University of Edinburgh
Nursing Studies Monographs

Nurse Teachers: The Report of an Opinion Survey
by A. Lancaster, M.Sc., MEd., R.G.N., S.C.M., R.N.T.

Patient-Nurse Interaction: A Study of Interaction
Patterns in Acute Psychiatric Wards
by Annie T. Altschul, B.A.(Lond.), M.Sc.(Edin.), S.R.N.,
R.M.N., R.N.T.

A Study of the Biological Sciences in Relation to Nursing

A Study of the Biological Sciences in Relation to Nursing

Kathleen J. W. Wilson
Ph.D., B.Sc., R.G.N., S.C.M., R.N.T.

Senior Research Fellow University of Birmingham and Nursing
    Research Liaison Officer, West Midlands Region.
Formerly Senior Lecturer, Department of Nursing Studies, University
of Edinburgh;
Examiner to the General Nursing Council for Scotland;
Principal Tutor, Preliminary Training School, Royal Infirmary,
Edinburgh;
Midwife, University College Hospital, London;
Nursing Sister, Colonial Nursing Service, Gold Coast.

CHURCHILL LIVINGSTONE
EDINBURGH LONDON AND NEW YORK 1975

CHURCHILL LIVINGSTONE
Medical Division of Longman Group Limited

Distributed in the United States of America by
Longman Inc., 72 Fifth Avenue, New York N.Y.
10011 and by associated companies, branches
and representatives throughout the world.

ISBN 0 443 01300 4

Library of Congress Cataloging in Publication Data
Wilson, Kathleen J W
    A study of the biological sciences in relation
to nursing
    Bibliography: p
    1.   Nurses and nursing — Study and teaching.
2.   Biology — Study and teaching. I. Title.
(DNLM: 1. Education, Nursing.   2. Biology — Education.
3.   Science — Education. WY18 W749b)
RT73.W54   331.1   75-4024

Printed in Great Britain

Preface

This report of a study of biological sciences in relation to nursing in adult medical and surgical wards is based on research which resulted in the submission of a thesis presented for the degree of Doctor of Philosophy in the Faculty of Social Sciences in the University of Edinburgh.

For various reasons beyond the control of the writer there was a considerable delay between the data collection in 1964 and the presentation of the thesis in 1971.

Because of the lapse of time between collecting the data and writing the report it was felt that some nursing practices included in the study might be outdated. In 1970 enquiries were made at the hospitals where the data were collected and it was found that the nursing activities studied were still being used, although it was not possible to find out how frequently or by which grades of nurse they were being carried out.

The system of references used in this thesis is a modified version of the Harvard System as described in *General Notes on the preparation of Scientific Papers* (The Royal Society, 1965). When two or more references are made to the same work, they are differentiated by the use of letters in the text (a, b . . .) which correspond to the letters and respective page numbers in the list of references.

With the exception of a few international publications, the reference material pertains only to Britain. Because of the substantial differences in the work of nurses and doctors and in the general and nursing education systems in other countries, any implied comparisons between conditions in Britain and those which exist elsewhere would have been inappropriate. Works relating to nursing in North America which provided background reading are listed in the bibliography, together with textbooks which were used in preparing the nurses' Science Test.

In general, nurses are referred to as female and doctors as male. The term 'ward sister' is used to represent the registered nurse in charge of a hospital ward and is intended to include her male counterpart, the charge nurse.

During the time this thesis was being written, the title 'Clinical Instructor' was changed to 'Clinical Teacher' *(The Nurses (Scotland) Rules 1970)*. The former term has been retained in the text.

Birmingham, 1975   K.J.W.W.

vii

Acknowledgments

I would like to express my thanks to everyone who helped to make this study possible, particularly to the late Miss Elsie Stephenson, who was Director of the Nursing Studies Unit, University of Edinburgh, when this study was started, for her supervision, interest and continual encouragement; to the late Professor R. Cruickshank for his valuable assistance as supervisor until he retired from the Chair of Bacteriology in the University of Edinburgh; to Professor S.L. Morrison, Department of Social Medicine, University of Edinburgh, for helpful advice during his period as supervisor; to Professor Margaret Scott Wright, Department of Nursing Studies, University of Edinburgh, for her supervision, encouragement and helpful criticism during the later stages of the study; to Professor H. J. Walton, Department of Psychiatry, University of Edinburgh, for his interest and advice at the beginning of this study and, later, for his valuable assistance and encouragement as supervisor; to Mr. J. Nimmo and the staff of the Research Centre for Social Sciences, University of Edinburgh, for their assistance with data processing; to the Scottish Home and Health Department, the South-Eastern Regional Hospital Board and the Boards of Management of the hospitals used in the study for permission to observe in the wards and for access to the samples of doctors and nurses; to the Matrons, Nurse Teachers and Ward Sisters who showed a lively interest in the study, and who provided facilities for observation in the wards and for the administration of tests to the nurses; to the Nurses and Patients in the wards, who so willingly accepted the presence of an observer; to the Nurses and Doctors who participated in the study; to the Staff and Students of the Department of Nursing Studies in the University of Edinburgh for their valuable comment on the questions being prepared for the nurses' Science Test and, more recently, for their helpful criticism of the research data; to Ames Company for a grant of £50 towards expenses incurred in the study.

1975

K.J.W.W.

Contents

List of Tables

List of Illustrations

Summary

The purpose of this study was to investigate: (i) the extent of staff nurses' knowledge of the biological sciences upon which nursing practices depend; (ii) the pattern of learning of these sciences during student nurse training; (iii) the extent to which staff and student nurses' knowledge of the biological sciences was related to the activities which they carried out in hospital wards and; (iv) the doctors' expectations of the staff nurses' knowledge and responsibilities.

A survey of the literature appeared to confirm the view that there was no clear definition of the extent of the knowledge of biological sciences required by practising registered nurses; that the employee status of student nurses prevented the effective coordination of theory and practice in their training programme; that appropriate criteria had not been established for selecting entrants to nursing. There was evidence that these factors have created problems in nursing education. In the practical situation, where the nursing and medical professions work in close cooperation, doctors have expressed conflicting opinions about the functions of registered nurses.

Methods

For purposes of the present study, three general hospitals were selected. An observation period of approximately 1800 hours was spent in two medical and two surgical wards in each hospital to record the frequency with which nursing activities were carried out respectively by staff nurses, third year, second year and first year students. The observed activities were used as the basis for an objective test designed to assess the nurses' knowledge of the biological sciences on which the activities depend.

A sample of 532 nurses was drawn from the three hospitals: 115 staff nurses, 136 third year, 143 second year and 138 first year students. They completed the Science Test and an intelligence test, and provided information about their general education.

A postal questionnaire, based on the same nursing activities, was completed by a sample of 179 doctors drawn from the same three hospitals. The doctors were asked to state whether they expected staff nurses to have the knowledge required by the Science Test, and whether they expected them to initiate and take responsibility for some of the activities.

Results

Comparison of the staff nurses' scores in the Science Test with results obtained from the Doctors' Questionnaire showed that the doctors expected staff nurses to have more knowledge than they displayed.

When items in the Science Test and in the Doctors' Questionnaire were classified according to the different biological sciences, no significant differences were found between staff nurses' scores and doctors' expectations.

When the total scores of the four groups of nurses in the Science Test were compared with each other, a significant increase was found with each year of seniority. When the scores of the groups were compared on each question, the greatest number of significant differences was found between first and second year students.

Comparison between the nurses' scores on items in the Science Test classified according to the different biological sciences showed no difference between the groups or between the sciences.

Correlation, for each group of nurses, between scores in the Science Test questions and the frequency with which each group carried out the associated activities showed that in one third of the questions correlations were + .60 or higher, in one third - .60 or higher, and in the remaining third indifferent or low.

The only consistently positive correlations between the nurses' scores in the Science Test and their general educational attainment were between combined Higher and Advanced level passes in any subject and the scores of nurses with passes at these levels.

A substantial positive correlation was found between the I.Q. and Science Test scores in each group of nurses.

Conclusions

It would seem that there is potential danger to patients in the discrepancy between the staff nurses' knowledge of biological sciences and the doctors' assumptions of their knowledge, as revealed in this study. To improve the registered nurses' knowledge, changes would probably be required in the system of nursing education.

On the basis of these findings, some suggestions have been made for changes which might improve the teaching of student nurses and the environment in which they receive their professional education.

The methods developed in this study could be modified and applied to other areas of nursing knowledge and used in schools of nursing to provide information on which to base the development and periodical revision of curricula.

1. Introduction

1.1 GENERAL BACKGROUND TO THE STUDY

The scientific theory upon which nursing depends is derived from two groups of disciplines. One is the behavioural sciences: psychology, sociology, social anthropology; the other the biological sciences: physiology, pharmacology, microbiology, anatomy. The behavioural sciences upon which nursing depends are excluded from consideration in the present study.

That there is a component of nursing which is based on a knowledge of the biological sciences has long been accepted by those responsible for nursing education. The statutory body, the General Nursing Council, has recognised this position by including these subjects in the syllabus of training and in both the written and the practical parts of the examination which leads to registration as a nurse.

The syllabus of training is stated in broad terms, consequently there is considerable variety in the range and depth of the biological science content of programmes in different schools.

No evidence has been found which provides a basis for the establishment of criteria regarding the standard of knowledge of the biological sciences required by the practising registered nurse. This lack of definition was expressed by the World Health Organization Regional Office for Europe in 1956 in the publication *Basic Nursing Curriculum in Europe:*

> As yet... the nursing profession as a whole is not sure as to the nature and extent of the scientific foundations which are essential. (a)

Earlier in the same work the need for a knowledge of the natural sciences was discussed:

> The natural sciences are needed to elucidate and illuminate nursing skills and techniques, many of which involve the use of complicated apparatus and modern scientific concepts. (b)

Beck (1958), while indicating the need for nurses to have a knowledge of the natural sciences, emphasised that the material taught should be selected because of its relevance to nursing:

> ... the natural sciences studied should form a basis for understanding the basic and technical nursing that make up the work of the nurse in hospital... There is a need to study in detail the fundamental principles of the natural and social sciences in relation to nursing and health care given, so that these subjects are not taught as ends in themselves but in order to inform and direct the work of the nurse.

Because there is no detailed information or advice available regarding the desirable range and depth of knowledge of the biological sciences which should be taught, nurse teachers have considerable freedom to decide what should be included in the programme. It is possible that in many schools the biological science content is considerably greater than the minimum which students require in order to pass the General Nursing Councils' examinations. The individual standards of the schools depend upon the nurses and doctors who participate in teaching and on the ability of the students to learn and to understand the material.

The part of nursing which is dependent on a knowledge of the biological sciences is probably more obviously affected by changes in medical sciences than are other aspects of nursing. The relationship between this aspect of nursing and medical practice highlights the need for continual adjustment of the nursing curriculum. With each change, the biological science content has to be identified and defined by the nurse teachers, and the role of nurses working in the wards has to be adjusted to accommodate new practices.

Attempts which have been made to define the role of the registered nurse have had to be stated in very general terms in order to encompass the wide variety of situations in which nursing is practised and the varied duties which nurses carry out.

The limitations of such definitions would seem to be twofold. Firstly, they may be stated in such general terms that they are of very little value in planning the curriculum for a school of nursing. Secondly, they have usually been formulated from within the nursing profession without regard for the expectations of others with whom nurses work. It is possible that some of these people, including the patients, have expectations regarding the role of nurses which are different from the nurses' image of their own role. In relation to patient care, the doctors constitute the professional group with whom nurses work most closely.

In the present study, the staff nurse group was chosen to represent professionally qualified nurses for two reasons. Firstly, they constitute the group of registered nurses who spend most time giving direct patient care. Secondly, because the majority of them are recently qualified, their knowledge of the biological sciences was unlikely to have increased greatly since they completed their training.

Doctors were included in this study because the care of patients depends to a large extent on the effective coordination of medical and nursing care. There is a close working relationship between doctors and staff nurses in hospital wards, particularly when the staff nurse is in charge in the absence of the ward sister. On such occasions the staff nurse deputises for the sister and accompanies the doctor when he visits patients and prescribes treatments. Having prescribed such treatments, doctors usually leave it to the nurse in charge to see that they are carried out. Doctors are not generally present in the wards continuously throughout the day and night and are therefore dependent on the nursing staff to observe and report any significant changes in the patients' medical and nursing condition. Since so much appears to depend upon nurses having the knowledge which enables them to carry out these responsibilities effectively, it seems reasonable to assume that doctors have certain expectations regarding the staff nurses' knowledge of the biological sciences.

Nursing activities may be classified into three groups:

a. activities which are carried out by nurses which are not normally prescribed by doctors, for example, care of the mouth, care of pressure areas;
b. activities prescribed by doctors and carried out by nurses, for example, administration of drugs, surgical dressings;
c. activities which doctors carry out themselves with the assistance of nurses, for example, abdominal paracentesis, lumbar puncture.

Some of the activities in group (a) may be prescribed by doctors for particular patients, for example, if a child has had a repair of cleft palate the mouth care would be prescribed by the surgeon who operated.

Individual doctors may vary in their ideas about the group to which an activity should be assigned. Their expectations of the nurses' knowledge may also vary according to how they would classify nursing activities and responsibilities.

1.1.1 General Plan of the study

The three groups of people involved are doctors, staff nurses and student nurses. As doctors and staff nurses are in close professional contact in the clinical situation, and as students spend a large proportion of their three year programme in giving nursing care, it was decided to base this study on nursing activities carried out in hospital wards.

The study is confined to the nursing care provided in adult medical and surgical wards. No account is taken of the timing and content of teaching of biological sciences in the schools of nursing.

The staff nurses' and student nurses' knowledge of the biological sciences related to certain nursing activities will be tested. The doctors will be asked about the knowledge they expect staff nurses to have in relation to some of these activities, and whether they expect them to initiate and take responsibility for others.

It was noted earlier that there is a lack of definition of the range and standard of knowledge of the biological sciences required by nurses.

By comparing the doctors' responses to these questions with the staff nurses' knowledge, the opinions of a closely related professional group may be used as a guide to the standard of knowledge of these sciences which is appropriate to the practising registered nurse.

By comparing the staff nurses' knowledge with that of the students, it may be possible to detect the pattern of learning which occurs throughout the three year educational programme.

The student nurses and staff nurses will be asked to complete an intelligence test and provide information about their levels of attainment in school subjects before entering nursing. It is planned to assess the relationship between these two factors and the nurses' knowledge of the biological sciences upon which nursing depends.

1.2 SOME INDICATIONS OF DOCTORS' EXPECTATIONS REGARDING NURSES AND NURSING

A review of the literature reveals sources of information which indicate, directly and indirectly, doctors' assumptions regarding the registered nurse's knowledge of biological sciences.

1.2.1 Direct expression of the doctors' expectations of the nurses' biological science knowledge can be found in textbooks and articles in nursing journals written by doctors for nurses.

The textbooks are addressed mainly to student nurses, although the authors sometimes suggest that the material could be of value to registered nurses.

It is not intended to present a systematic review of, or to comment on, the level of knowledge which the doctor expects the student to have acquired by the end of her training. This would require a separate research project not within the scope of this study. However, the following impressions were gained from reading a number of textbooks:

1. Where an introductory review of anatomy and physiology is presented before the medical and surgical conditions are dealt with, the level of presentation frequently varies in different parts of the same text. It may be that the sections which deal with the topics of special interest to the physician or surgeon receive special attention, or that the writer has had the experience of lecturing and examining student nurses and has found that he has had to supplement their knowledge in these areas of anatomy and physiology before going on to deal with the pathology and treatment of disease.

2. Descriptions of signs and symptoms and the aims of medical treatment of individual diseases would seem to be at a fairly consistent level throughout a text. The background pathology appears to be presented when it has obvious relevance to nursing observations. The writers presumably know that nurses who have a special interest in a topic, and who wish to study it in greater depth, have access to medical textbooks. These are available in the nursing school libraries.

3. The titles of texts written by doctors for nurses often provide a valuable guide to their contents. They indicate that their purpose is to present a medical specialty to a nursing audience, e.g. medicine for nurses, surgery for nurses, gynaecology for nurses. The writers are quite specifically *not* presenting nursing textbooks.

The doctors who write articles for nursing journals are obviously medical specialists who feel that it would be to the advantage of patients, nurses and doctors if nurses who were caring for patients with a specific complaint had a greater depth of knowledge. It would seem that some of the articles are written for the nurse who is about to go to an area of practice which requires some highly specialised knowledge, for example, a coronary care unit, a surgical neurology unit, etc. Only a few of the articles read gave guidance on what and what not to do without explaining why.

1.2.2 Indirect expression of the doctors' expectations of the nurses' knowledge of the biological sciences are to be found in the medical journals. These take the form of statements which are indicative of the attitudes of doctors to nurses and to nursing, but rarely make direct reference to the biological sciences.

Most of the discussion revolves around the changes in the role of the nurse which the doctor would like to see implemented. As nurses work closely with doctors, it is perhaps understandable that the suggested changes are invariably associated with developments in the organisation and the practice of medicine. Only a few of the comments refer to changes which are deprecated by the doctor and which he would like to prevent. In none of the material consulted was there any direct reference to the need for nurses to have an adequate knowledge of the biological sciences in order to carry out effectively the activities which are consistent with her role, as it is seen by the doctor.

The opinions expressed are associated with a wide variety of situations.

1.2.2.1 *Team leadership: different degrees of involvement of doctors and nurses with patients.* The doctor regards himself as the leader of the ward team even although he spends a very limited period of time in the ward each day. Conran (1970) made the comment that doctors rarely expose themselves to the conscious patient for more than 'an hour in the day—indeed it is doubtful if it commonly attains an hour in the week'.

However, all the other members of the ward team are involved with caring for the patients whose admission to the ward can only be sanctioned by the doctor. He chooses the patient with whom he and the other team members work. Conran (1970) enumerates the choices which the doctor has in relation to the patient and the limitations placed on the nurse:

> There is, in every doctor's encounter with a patient, some freedom of choice. There is the freedom of the general practitioner to choose to refer his patient to a specialist. He has a second choice in selecting the specialist. The specialist is primarily selective in his choice of specialty, secondly in his manner of disposal... The consultant retains a further range of choice—to change his mind. It requires but a moment to realise that the nurse in hospital has, except within a very limited working range, no such comparable freedom to choose. She must accept, and relate to, a personality chosen for her, and to implement treatment as directed.

The work which the nurse does in relation to each patient is inevitably circumscribed by the diagnostic and therapeutic aims of the doctor in charge of the patient. However, using the classification of nursing activities which was described above (1.1) it can be seen that many of the nursing activities which are carried out in the wards are not prescribed by the doctor. It is possible that he would only know about these activities if they were not carried out.

1.2.2.2 *Paternal Attitude.* The idea of the doctor as the leader of the ward team is probably influenced by the paternalistic attitude of the members of a largely male profession and the fact that nursing is a mainly female profession. This is dealt with at some length by Conran (1970) where he says:

> The triangular relationship between doctor, nurse and patient thus contrived to define roles quite clearly, paralleling the earlier father-mother-child relationship whence the patient had come, and back into which his illness drove him.

The common use of the possessive pronoun by doctors when they are discussing nursing staff and patients serves to emphasise their paternalistic attitude towards those with whom they work. This is demonstrated in the article by Conran, quoted above, and by the anonymous author of 'The Paediatrician' in the *British Medical Journal* (1970):

> When the junior staff changed over there was inevitably a period when there was no one with practical experience of emergencies in neonates and young babies. It was at times like this that ward sisters were invaluable. All my sisters know they can phone me if they are concerned about a baby...

1.2.2.3 *The Organisation of nursing as it affects the work of the doctor.* The working relationships between doctors and nurses in the actual ward situation are, on the whole, congenial. It is in this situation that the care of individual patients is the first priority. The cooperation and understanding between the two groups are most evident when an emergency arises, when they work together in close cooperation to do the best that can be done for the patient, unconcerned about professional differentiation.

Expressions of the doctors' attitudes to nursing and nurses are to be found when they take a longer view of the situation. Doctors have limited knowledge of the sum total of activities which are involved in providing a nursing service for 24 hours a day, seven days a week. It is, therefore, not surprising that their comments about nursing and nurses tend to be related to the effects which the practice of nursing has on the practice of medicine.

Bowers (1970), in an article entitled 'Why not Teach Nursing to Doctors?', says:

> Another aspect of nursing which is a closed book to many doctors is the *routine* of a ward. Any doctor who is interested enough to comment on the policy of the unit should

make it his business to know about change lists, meal times... the daily nursing report... the duties of the theatre sister, and so on.

There are indications that changes in the organisation of nursing services and in the preparation of nurses, when seen to affect the nursing service situation, is viewed with some concern by doctors. There are occasional nostalgic references to the ward sister of the past, such as Sir George Pickering's (1971) comment in his address entitled 'Medicine and Society—Past, Present and Future' delivered on the occasion of the opening of the new Medical School at Nottingham:

What made British nurses the envy of the world was the ward sister and her senior staff. Intelligent, dedicated, kindly women worked long hours and saw to the physical and mental comfort of the patients entrusted to them, cooperating with doctors in their treatment. When I was at St. Mary's two ward sisters were, in my opinion, much better diagnosticians than any of my colleagues. I profitted (sic) many times by their advice. This has changed and is changing for the worse... The real reason is quite simple, nurses *qua* nurses are not valued as they should be. They are, and always have been, badly paid, and they have not always been treated with the great respect that is their due.

Attempts to improve their status have taken two wrong directions. One, in which the United States has led, has been to take them in training from the wards into the lecture theatres and even chemistry laboratories, to stuff their minds with what that great educator and philosopher, Arthur Whitehead,* called the tyranny of inert ideas. A remark of Whitehead's is apt, "Uneducated clever women... are in middle life so much the most cultured part of the community. They have been saved from the horrible burden of inert ideas".

Undoubtedly there are exceptional people who can function at the level described by Sir George, who have a minimum of formal education in nursing, but it is questionable whether the numbers of nurses required to take responsible positions in the National Health Service could be provided from this source.

1.2.2.4 *The age of ward sisters.* It would seem that the age of the nurse has a significant influence on her status, in the eyes of some writers. In his description of the ward sister Sir George Pickering appears to be thinking of a middle aged woman. An editorial in the *Lancet* (1971), on the 'Teaching of Asepsis to Students', seems to be an expression of regret at the passing of

the senior ward sisters, who used to regiment the surgical dressers

and of concern about their

replacement by younger women... who cannot try to teach surgical techniques to medical students without some loss of face for the students.

It would seem that the ward sister is only acceptable as a teacher of medical personnel if she cannot be classified as young. There is no reference here to her professional knowledge and expertise.

*Whitehead, Alfred North, (1963). *The Aims of Education*, p.13. New York: Macmillan.

1.2.2.5 *The clinical responsibilities of nurses.* Sir George Pickering
(1971) obviously believed that the ward sister was capable of a
considerable degree of sophistication as a diagnostician; however, there
is no evidence in his address that he would be prepared to give formal
recognition to this as a function of the nurse. On the other hand, there
are writers who express the view that nurses are capable of taking more
clinical responsibility than they are given at present. In relation to the
staffing of casualty departments, Burkett (1970) says that a doctor

> may be totally inexperienced, come from some remote foreign medical school whose
> training is different from ours, have only spent a minimal time in Britain, and may only
> speak a smattering of English. This, however, is medico-legally more acceptable than that
> the patient be seen by a fully competent sister with many years of casualty experience in
> this country behind her—surely an absurd state of affairs?
>
> We are constantly giving lip service to improvement of the status of the nursing
> profession. We change their names, we change their uniforms, we change their pay, but as
> soon as it comes to giving them clinical responsibility—surely the acid test of our opinion
> of their worth—we hold up our hands in horror.

Doctors' attitudes towards nurses seem to be varied and sometimes
contradictory. Their knowledge of a nurse's work is necessarily limited
and many are reluctant to see her in any role other than as the provider
of direct patient care. The idea implicit in the recommendations of the
Committee on Senior Nursing Staff Structure, that she should develop
her managerial, decision-making role, has been questioned by members
of the medical profession.

However, although nurses' clinical expertise is generally recognised,
the knowledge which she requires in order to fulfil her role as it is seen by
her medical colleagues is nowhere clearly defined and has possibly not
been identified. In view of the limited amount of theory which a nurse is
taught during her basic training, much of her knowledge has to be
'picked up' in the clinical situation, both during her training and
subsequently as a qualified, practising nurse. This time-consuming
method of acquiring knowledge is perhaps responsible for the
importance placed upon 'seniority', both by doctors and within the
nursing profession itself. It does at least provide senior nurses with a
means of preserving their traditional position of authority.

1.2.2.6 *Relationships of general practitioners with health visitors vis-à-
vis social workers.* Considerable interest has been shown by general
practitioners in the role and functions of the health visitor. Their
attitudes to health visitors emerged in discussions regarding the
functions of social workers which followed the publication of the
(Seebohm) *Report of the Committee on Local Authority and Allied
Personal Services* (Home Department, 1968). Some doctors appeared
to be uncertain about the role, functions and education of the social
workers and preferred to rely on the established health visitor. This was
evident in a leading article in the *British Medical Journal* (1970). After

commenting on the precipitate manner in which the social work acts had been passed the writer went on to say:

> There is, of course, a shortage of social workers as their is of doctors and nurses. The standards of qualification in nursing and medicine are well defined, long established, and recognized by a public which has the protection of the General Nursing and General Medical Councils. Social workers are still establishing their discipline, and there might have been less opposition from doctors to the Seebohm proposals if the intention had been to introduce them gradually and when there were enough qualified, trained, and experienced social workers available.

This implied that the public ought to be protected from the ministrations of social workers until a statutory body is formed to oversee their standards of education and practice. It is interesting to note that the qualifications of other professions supplementary to medicine, for example, physiotherapists, radiographers, dietitians, occupational therapists, appear to have been accepted by doctors before their professional education and standards of practice were controlled by statute. It was not until 1960 that the Professions Supplementary to Medicine Act was passed, after which boards were set up to provide this control.

Sim (1970), in a comment on social workers vis-à-vis health visitors, indicates that there is a considerable amount of anxiety about the preparation and role of social workers in psychiatric practice. Again, the writer prefers to work with the known health visitor:

> Once upon a time there were few social workers, but now they have proliferated to such an extent that they are usurping the role of the doctor at all levels. If it were shown that they had the necessary skills and were effective in their allotted tasks one would have to concede that for the sake of progress these changes must be. But there is not a shred of evidence that this is so... Their roles may be defined, but they have not yet been established, and one would have thought before increasing the size of our social services, providing career structures, and giving social workers authority over doctors, one would have investigated what they are capable of doing and what it costs and compare cost and efficiency with alternative methods.
>
> A year ago I decided to experiment and took on two trained nurses who were health visitors in a neighbouring borough. After three months' attendance at our inpatient and day hospital units with a planned course of instruction, they were more competent in dealing with material degrees of psychiatric disability in the community than a recently qualified psychiatric social worker, even though their educational attainments were less. Of even greater importance, they could effectively carry a larger case load.

It would seem that doctors are wary of social workers because their professional role and standards of practice have not been clearly defined. They prefer working with nurses because they know, or think they know, the extent of a nurse's knowledge and feel that they can depend upon her as a co-worker.

It is interesting to note that an editorial in the *British Medical Journal* should suggest, by inference, that nurses have established their discipline. The fact that many nurses are themselves doubtful about this was one of the reasons for carrying out the present study.

1.2.2.7 *Attachment of health visitors and district nurses to general practices, with emphasis on the work of district nurses.* In the past decade changes have occurred, and are continuing to occur, in the working arrangements between the family doctors and community nursing services. During this period an increasing number of health visitors and district nurses have been 'attached' to general practices. There is a variety of types and degrees of 'attachment' but all of these necessitate the development of a closer working relationship between the two professional groups. Anderson and Draper (1967) described the different types of attachment and liaison. In some cases the doctors have employed a 'practice nurse'; in others, nurses employed by the local health authority have been assigned to work with the doctors in a particular group practice. In both cases there has been a considerable change in the actual work, and in the organisation of the work, of both nurses and doctors. Lord (1965) expressed something of the attitudes of the doctors to these changes when he said:

> The differing policies regarding health visitor attachment originates within the differing philosophies and personalities of the nursing and medical professions and the profession as a whole must begin to think more in terms of general-practitioner-directed health visiting, and less about routine health visitor visiting which could ultimately be dropped...
>
> Fears are often expressed that the health visitor might become an assistant to the general practitioner instead of being a professional worker in her own right. I feel she should become an extension of his own service, and the universal attachment of health visitors can only be seen as a means of grafting new life and interest into this branch of the profession whose evolution and progressive improvement have been so pot-bound since the 1948 Health Act... Experience has invariably shown that where health visitors are already working with general practitioners both find their work enriched and their relationship improved and their usefulness increased.

Lord did not discuss district nurses in his article. However, Boddy (1969a), in his study *The General Practitioner's View of the Home Nursing Service*, sought the opinions of 500 doctors selected at random from the list of 'Doctors providing General Medical Services' of all the Executive Councils in Scotland. He found that:

> half the respondents considered that the present work of the District Nursing Sister does not make best use of her professional training and skills.*

This confirms the findings of Carstairs (1966) and Hockey (1966).

Boddy (1969b) found that although 'only 13% of the respondents had District Nursing Sisters attached to their practice organisation', 71% of the remainder said that they would like such an attachment.

Weston Smith and Mottram (1967) and Weston Smith and O'Donovan (1970) describe their experience of having a nurse, employed by the practice, working with the general practitioners. In the former paper they say that:

*'Present work' in this context refers to the work of district nurses who are not 'attached' to general medical practices.

It was thought that the scope of [doctors] work, both in hospital and in the care of greater numbers of patients, could be done efficiently and properly provided that time was not wasted with minor problems, especially unnecessary visiting and revisiting and routine procedures in the surgery.

In a publication by the Royal College of General Practitioners (1968), *The Practice Nurse*, this view is substantiated. It was felt that there were considerable difficulties in making accurate quantitative estimates of the time which is saved by the doctor in having a nurse attached to the practice. However:

> The overall impression of the doctors is that the advent of the nurse resulted in a saving of time which enabled the doctors to practice (sic) medicine at a level which they had been unable to reach previously. Whilst their work was as demanding as before, they enjoyed it much more and were less aware of fatigue. This was attributed to the degree of work satisfaction which was achieved.

The doctors quoted above seemed confident, as did those who commented on the work of ward sisters, that they knew the extent of the nurses' capabilities. And yet, here again, the nurses' competence must to a large extent depend on their own ability to continue to develop their professional knowledge beyond the limitations of formal training.

1.2.2.8 *The transfer to nurses of activities in patient care which doctors formerly considered to be their prerogative.* The question of 'who does what' in relation to the investigation of patients, the assessment of their condition, and the treatments prescribed by doctors, has long been debated by nurses and doctors. This question has become more pertinent with the rapid development of the technology which now plays a large part in the practice of medicine and nursing. Some writers feel that nurses have not been able to keep pace with the technological advances in medicine. Conran (1970) says:

> Doctors know more and know better, and nurses can no longer speak their language.

This view is supported in a leading article entitled 'Doctor and nurse' in the *Lancet* (1970):

> With increasing technology in the hospital, the gap between the doctor's knowledge and that of the nurse has widened... One solution is to train the nurse to a high degree of technical competence.

There is no suggestion that nurses should 'know more and know better'.

Considerable difficulties are encountered when attempting to define which activities should be carried out by doctors and which by nurses. These were recognised in the report published by the Nuffield Provincial Hospitals Trust (1953a) on *The Work of Nurses in Hospital Wards* where the writer explains that:

> The procedures which are performed by nurses and those which are regarded as the prerogative of the doctor are by no means clearly defined and the accepted policy of one hospital does not necessarily correspond with that of another.

Later, Scott (1965), taking a broader view of medical and social services provided by a variety of different workers, drew attention to the constantly changing situation in which the

line of demarcation between medical and social care is never sharp or absolute and is certainly not constant... It changes with changes in medical knowledge and medical practice as our own professional horizons expand or shrink.

It would seem that there is no clear line between medical and nursing practice—in fact there would appear to be a considerable area of overlap. From the variety of opinions expressed and systems in operation, it would seem that any attempt to establish rigid lines of demarcation could be to the detriment of the patients.

The stages through which an activity passes before it becomes an accepted part of the practice of nursing are of some interest. There appears to be a sequence of events associated with the introduction of activities in patient care which are based on advances in medical knowledge and technology. In the teaching hospitals in particular, an activity is usually introduced on an experimental basis, using equipment which is at the prototype stage of development. In view of this situation, it is understandable that doctors wish to carry out the experiment themselves. The result may be that the activity is abandoned, or that the equipment is further developed and refined. When a stage of refinement is reached, which leads to the production of a piece of standardised equipment, and the results of its use are predictable, the doctors may feel sufficiently confident to ask the nurse to take over the activity.

Another factor which may influence the passing of an activity from doctor to nurse is the frequency with which the activity is prescribed, for example, with the advance in knowledge of the significance of changes in patients' blood pressure, particularly after surgery, doctors prescribed blood pressure readings at fifteen and thirty minute intervals. In view of the fact that the medical staff were usually still working in the operating theatre at this time, these frequent blood pressure readings became an accepted part of the nursing care of the patient after operation.

The rapid changes in nursing practice which have been precipitated by technological developments are highlighted in a leading article in the *British Medical Journal* (1967) on 'Resuscitation and the Nurse':

The report... of the latest meeting of the Joint Committee of the British Medical Association and the Royal College of Nursing illustrates the rapidly evolving role of the nurse in the changing medical scene. Within the memory of senior members of the profession student nurses were not expected to take the blood pressure or give intramuscular injections. Now they must understand intermittent positive-pressure respirators and cardiac monitors, apparently give intravenous injections, and even undertake the onerous responsibility of initiating treatment of cardiac arrest.

When nurses are asked to take over an activity which has previously been carried out by doctors there is usually a considerable amount of discussion and diversity of opinion expressed as to whether the change should be made. In recent years discussion has revolved around a number of topics, including the administration of drugs by the intravenous route, the suturing of the perineum by midwives, and the paying of first visits to patients in their homes by nurses attached to general practices.

At a joint meeting of the Royal College of Nursing and the British Medical Association *(British Medical Journal*, 1967, 'Nurses and Doctors') the Royal College of Nursing seemed to be reluctant to accept that nurses should give drugs by the intravenous route. It would seem, from the tone of the statement which was issued, that they were under considerable pressure from the British Medical Association to accept this as a nursing practice. The statement read:

> The R.C.N. policy is that the giving of intravenous drugs by nurses, even when the needle was in situ, is not a normal nursing duty. However, the College accepted that with certain safeguards nurses might exceptionally undertake this task if it was necessary in order to maintain the service to the patient. The Committee endorsed the view of its Chairman (Mr A. Staveley Gough) to the effect that a registered nurse could administer drugs by the intravenous route provided that the intravenous needle or catheter had been inserted by a doctor and that the nurse concerned had received full instruction from the medical staff on the methods to be used; and that in such circumstances the medical staff must take responsibility for any accident or complication which might arise unless it was due to any negligence on the part of the nurse—for example, if she gave the wrong drug or the wrong dose of a drug.

This subject was again discussed in a leading article in the *Lancet* (1970) in relation to the addition of drugs to an intravenous infusion. After discussing the dangers of adding drugs to infusions and the danger of the drug undergoing chemical change when exposed to light or when mixed with the infusion fluid, the writer went on to say:

> All drugs given by nurses [into intravenous infusions] should be precisely prescribed on suitable forms, complex mixtures should be avoided, and drugs should not normally be added to blood... Another precaution is the training of nurses to give drugs into drip tubing...

In both of these examples, training is referred to in terms of the acquisition of technical skills. There is no mention of possible complications and of the need for close observation of the patient after the injection to detect any abnormal reaction which might occur.

There has been a considerable amount of discussion and study of the work of nurses attached to general practices. The activity which has proved to be most controversial has been related to the nurse paying first visits to patients in their homes.

Weston Smith and Mottram (1967) and Weston Smith and O'Donovan (1970) have described in considerable detail the work of the nurse attached to their practice. They have built what they consider to be adequate safeguards into their system of working. In the former article they say:

> We think that the modern nurse is in a position to assess whether a patient is ill enough to need the visit of a doctor; in other words, we are placing her in the position of a sister with a responsible hospital position.

A contrary view was expressed by Marsh (1969):

Smith and Mottram (1967) described how their nurse visited all patients who asked for a call and selected those she considered that the doctor needed to see; she appeared to be working, firstly, as a diagnostician of the gravity of illness, and, secondly, as a therapist of those illnesses for which she thought consultation by a doctor was not necessary... the medical climate of opinion in our practice did not favour such a radical innovation.

Bird (1968) expresses more forcibly Marsh's reservations about nurses paying first visits in general practice, then goes on to enumerate what he considers she should do:

If a nurse is asked to diagnose and initiate treatment she is doing the work of a doctor... The skill of the general practitioner is above all else in distinguishing and diagnosing through history and physical signs the important from the unimportant symptoms. A nurse cannot do this. But a nurse in the practice can do all the routine work which enables a doctor to use his skill... In our practice she runs the inoculation programme, takes the swabs, urine, blood, etc., both at home and in the surgery, gets them 'written up' and dealt with—does E.S.Rs., takes and mounts E.C.G. tracings, records the peak flow measurements, sets up pelvic traction for those with prolapsed intravertebral discs at home, visits the elderly and chronic sick (alternating with the doctor) and occasionally follows up from first visits, taking blood and other tests as needed...

It will be a great pity if excessive demands reduce the practice nurse to the role of a 'feldsher', when, losing the confidence of the public, general practice as we know it today will disintegrate.

The extremes of opinion expressed in these examples are of interest. Weston Smith and Mottram consider that nurses paying first visits to patients in their homes is a responsibility which is comparable with that of the ward sister. Marsh and Bird, on the other hand, clearly indicate that they consider this the work of the doctor. In none of these examples is there mention of the knowledge of the biological sciences which the nurse would require in order to function in this way.

Bird enumerates some activities which are not normally included in the nurse's curriculum, but no mention is made of the preparation which she would require in order to carry out these activities.

It would seem that the doctors' assumptions about a nurse's knowledge are of particular importance when there is any question of transferring to nurses an activity previously carried out by a doctor to overestimate a nurse's knowledge. Nurses may not know what they do not know.

The list of activities which has been discussed is by no means exhaustive. It is, however, representative of those which have been under discussion in recent years. Comments on the preparation of the nurse to undertake activities which are prescribed by the doctor have been, with a few exceptions, confined to ensuring their technical competence.

Writers who refer to the doctor's dependence on the nurse for accurate observation of, and reporting on, the patients' condition, rarely concern themselves with the nurses' understanding of the aims and possible complications of the treatments which have been prescribed.

It would seem that technical skill, and skill in making informed observation and in reporting, are separate and different accomplishments. It is around this difference that much of the controversy and confusion about nursing education revolves.

The former refers to the manual dexterity which some people can acquire through practice, after having been shown how to carry out an activity. This competence does not necessitate an understanding of the possible effects of the treatment, or of the scientific principles upon which the activity is based. The latter requires an understanding of the aims and objectives of medical prescription and a theoretical knowledge of the biological sciences upon which the activity, and its effects on the patient, depend.

The writers cited above mention the training needs of the nurse in terms of the instruction which she requires in order to acquire the necessary manual dexterity and technical skills. This emphasis is also demonstrated by Arthure (1970), Chairman of the Central Midwives Board, in a letter to the *British Medical Journal* where he explains the views of the Board on the subject of midwives suturing the perineum:

> It is the view of the Board that midwives who have been taught the technique of repairing the perineum, and are judged to be competent, may be authorized by the doctor concerned to carry out this procedure; the final responsibility will rest with the doctor.

Another example is to be found in a discussion on the views of the Scottish general practitioners on the preparation of nurses to work in attachment schemes in which Boddy (1969c) stated:

> The adequacy of general training, of course, leaves aside the question of whether or not the nurse would require training in the specific techniques associated with particular activities.

This rather narrow view of the preparation of the nurse may be due to the doctor's experience during their own preparation for medical practice, in which they have had an extensive theoretical preparation followed by a period of clinical practice before being registered by the General Medical Council. The academic preparation of the doctor, in addition to providing him with an advanced level of theoretical knowledge, provides him with an opportunity to apply the scientific method to medical practice. Because much of the material which is used for teaching is based on research findings, he realises that his education does not stop when he is registered by the General Medical Council. It may be that the doctor assumes that nursing education has provided the nurse with similar opportunities and that the addition of a new technique to her repertoire will be supported by scientific knowledge which she will supplement by further study if this should be necessary.

The impressions gained from these comments made by doctors about nurses and nursing would seem to indicate that doctors feel confident that they know the work which nurses are capable of undertaking. They appear to assume that changes and developments in medical care and in the organisation of medical practice should be accompanied by appropriate changes in nursing practice and that, when nurses have learned a skill which is new to them, they will have or will acquire the knowledge which will enable them to carry it out effectively.

1.3 STAFF NURSES AND STUDENT NURSES: THE SITUATION IN HOSPITAL WARDS

1.3.1 Introduction

As indicated above, staff nurses were selected to represent registered nurses in the present study. It was felt that they could provide information about the level of knowledge of the biological sciences which might be expected in newly qualified nurses and that doctors, through working closely with them, were likely to have expectations about their knowledge of the biological sciences.

Staff nurses are the product of a three-year nursing education programme during which, as students, they have spent approximately 120 weeks practising nursing in hospital wards and departments, and a minimum of 24 weeks in classroom study.

During the period of classroom study the students are taught the theory associated with nursing, according to the nurse teachers' interpretation of the syllabus of training provided by the General Nursing Council.

The fact that the syllabus is stated in broad terms makes it possible for the nursing school staff to adapt its content to incorporate material associated with changes in nursing practice. In relation to the biological science content of the students' programme, changes are likely to result from the effects on nursing of changes and developments in medical practice.

In the ward situation students occupy a dual role. They are nominally students of the school of nursing while at the same time they are employed by the Hospital Boards of Management as nursing service personnel. As a result of their occupation of this dual role, their education in the wards takes second place to the nursing service which they provide.

Because student nurses spend such a large part of their training period in giving nursing service it was decided to include them in the present study. It was felt that comparisons of the students' knowledge at different stages in their programme would provide some indications of the pattern of learning of the biological sciences associated with the nursing activities which they carry out in the wards.

Over the past three decades many writers have drawn attention to the fact that student nurses do not have a planned programme of nursing practice related to the teaching of the biological sciences, or to the teaching of any of the other sciences, on which nursing practice depends. Students have been allocated to clinical areas by nursing service administrators, and the immediate demands of nursing service have inevitably taken precedence over long-term educational needs.

Where such a situation exists, there are obvious difficulties in deciding how and when student nurses should be taught the theoretical background of the activities which they are expected to carry out, in defining the area of scientific knowledge appropriate to these activities, and in relating theory to practice in a way which is meaningful to the student.

In order to appreciate the findings of the present study, it is necessary to consider some of the conditions under which student nurses obtain their professional experience.

1.3.2 Nursing staff in hospital wards

There is no standard pattern of staffing in hospital wards. It varies in different hospitals, and in different wards within the same hospital. The duties of each category of nurse may be different in different places and, even in the same place, may be different at different times.

A ward is normally in charge of a ward sister. Below, there are five grades of nursing personnel who may be used to make up the nursing team:

a. staff nurses, who have completed a three-year training programme and are registered nurses;

b. student nurses, who may be at any stage of their three-year preparation for registration;

c. enrolled nurses, who have completed a two-year practical nursing programme, and would not normally be expected to take charge of a ward;

d. pupil nurses, who may be at any stage of their two-year preparation for enrolment;

e. auxiliaries (orderlies) who have had a variable amount of in-service training, depending on the provisions for training which are available in individual hospitals.

The ward staffing situation is made more complex by the fact that many staff nurses, enrolled nurses and auxiliaries work part-time and, in a few hospitals, pupil nurses also work and train on a part-time basis.

Within this complex of staff, it is often difficult for student nurses to know what is expected of them; for example, in the absence of a registered nurse, a problem may arise as to who is in charge of a ward if a third year student and an enrolled nurse are on duty at the same time. Owing to the wide range of ability among nurses and students, the formal question of 'seniority' may be less important in the care of the patients than the ability of the individual chosen to take charge of the ward.

The instability of the staffing structure may result in a student, or indeed a staff nurse, finding herself in a junior position one day, and on the next day in a position of considerable responsibility.

The Oxford Area Nurse Training Committee (1966a), in its report *From Student to Nurse*, discusses the situation in the wards where seniority and responsibility are defined in the following terms:

The range and nature of technical skills demanded of junior and senior nurses differs widely and ward work can be arranged, at least in theory, in a hierarchical order ranging from work which requires little or no skill to work which requires the greatest skill of which a nurse is deemed capable. When senior staff talk about the senior student nurse's position as having 'responsibility' they are defining responsibility in this second sense [in terms of technical skill].

The same report goes on to say that students

...have to come to terms with the fact that, though in theory progression in the hierarchy of skills depends on length of training, there are all sorts of factors in the nursing situation in reality, such as staff shortage, sickness and different attitudes towards training held by different ward sisters, which prevent the strict equation of the position held in the hierarchy with the stage of training. Because of staff shortages a senior student may be required to carry out some task which belongs properly to the position of a junior nurse. This may be and frequently is, interpreted as a loss of status. The position is particularly acute for the second year nurse who may be the equivalent of a senior in one ward and then fall to the equivalent of a junior at the next ward change.

The frequently changing role of the student nurses was described by the Nuffield Provincial Hospitals Trust (1953b) in their report of a job analysis:

It is clear that any shortage of trained nurses will immediately affect the position of the senior student nurses, whose status in the ward hierarchy will thereby be raised... Moreover, even the junior student is affected in that the scope of work for which she is responsible may be widened, while at the same time there can be less supervision of it by trained staff.

The staff nurses may also find that their role changes from day to day. When the ward sister is off duty they deputise for her; when she is on duty, they are expected to undertake a wide variety of activities, depending upon which other grades of staff are available.

In such a situation, the student nurse is faced with a kind of three-dimensional insecurity. As far as the patients are concerned, she knows only too well that she lacks the knowledge and experience which are required to cope with all the demands which they make upon her. There is little stability in the nursing team of which she is a member and yet, as a student, she must constantly depend on other members of the group for help and advice. Her own role is poorly defined and frequently changes. In such a situation, it is difficult to envisage how a planned and progressive learning programme could be organised or achieved.

1.3.3 The status of student nurses in the hospital environment

1.3.3.1 *The dual role of student and employee.* Student nurses occupy a dual role in the hospital ward situation. They are employees of the Boards of Management which administer the hospital service, and they are also students undertaking a three-year preparation for registration by the General Nursing Council.

At the time when the data for the present study were collected, student nurses in Scotland were required by the General Nursing Council to spend a minimum of 24 weeks in classroom study. The remainder of their training, approximately 120 weeks, was spent in nursing practice carried out in hospital wards and departments. In addition, the Council specified the number of weeks of practice which the students should have in different clinical areas, for example, in medical wards, surgical wards, operating theatres and out-patient departments. By means of information provided by its Inspector of Training Schools, the General Nursing Council approved (or disapproved) the clinical training areas used by each school of nursing. In this way the Council established, and to some extent controlled, the standard of the students' physical environment and of the equipment which was available for their use during clinical practice.

However, the General Nursing Council did not stipulate the number of weeks which a student should spend in a particular ward. This was decided by the nursing administrators in the hospital and was dependent on service needs. As a result, a student could spend three or four months in, for instance, a medical ward, or she may gain her experience of medical nursing by spending a short period in a number of different medical wards. Either situation could have disadvantages for the student, but the trend seems to have changed. In the *Report of the Working Party on the Recruitment and Training of Nurses* (1947a), issued jointly by the Ministry of Health, the Department of Health for Scotland and the Ministry of Labour and National Service, it was stated that:

...a student nurse who is compelled to remain in the same ward under the same sister for an unduly long period is apt to lose interest and may abandon her training altogether.

In 1970, the General Nursing Council for Scotland found it necessary to stipulate that student nurses should not spend less than eight weeks in any one ward or department. However, changes in the student nurses' programme, in terms of the variety of clinical practice and the length of time spent in different clinical areas, has not changed the status of the students. They are still expected to fill the dual role of student and employee. The Boards of Management, who are responsible for providing a hospital nursing service, delegate their authority as employers to senior nursing service administrators who, working in close liaison with nursing school staff, take the responsibility of employing and discharging student nurses. The nursing service administrators are obliged to rely to a very large extent upon student nurses to supply the nursing service needs of their hospitals, albeit within the broad framework of the General Nursing Council's requirements.

Crichton and Crawford (1966), discussing the responsibilities of hospital matrons in relation to nurse training schools, stated that:

At the moment, of course, the Matron is officially the head of the training school and the Principal Nurse Tutor holds no final responsibility.

With some exceptions, the same situation still seems to exist today. In accordance with the provisions of the *Report of the Committee on Senior Nursing Staff Structure*, issued jointly in 1966 by the Ministry of Health and the Scottish Home and Health Department, the senior post in the nursing hierarchy is the Chief Nursing Officer. She is responsible for the Teaching Division(s) within the group and for nursing service in one or more hospitals.

The students' training allowance and the hours which they work are established by the Nurses and Midwives Whitley Council. Their hours per week are the same as for fully qualified staff and their training allowancee is graduated so that they receive an increment each year. Deductions made at source from their training allowance include income tax and contributions toward superannuation, national insurance and the graduated pension scheme.

The conflict and dissatisfaction which has resulted from this joint employee/student role has long been a subject of comment in reports and in studies of nursing.

The point of view of the hospital authorities was clearly expressed in their evidence to the Lancet Commission (1932). They indicated that the work and discipline within nursing service would be at risk if students were allowed to pay fees:

If it is remembered that the main preoccupation of a hospital, in connexion with staffing, is to provide an adequate and stable nursing service for the patients, it is no paradox that the employment of student labour on a salary basis has advantages which would be lacking were the student allowed to pay actual fees for her training. These advantages turn on: (1) stability of labour force, (2) maintenance of the supply of candidates, (3) discipline, and (4) discouragement of complaints.

...The maintenance of discipline would, it is held, be difficult if the staff consisted mainly of unpaid, fee-paying students. They would not regard themselves as the employees of the hospital, but as students rendering voluntary service. The hospitals, for the most part, prefer, therefore, to pay the whole of their staffs, and to make training incidental to employment. That the pay is less than it would be were no training given does not alter the status of employee, which it is convenient to the hospital to retain.

The lack of provision for her instruction in the wards and the quality of her lectures and classes might, in some hospitals, be criticised by a probationer who was paying fees for her training.

In spite of the fact that the members of the Lancet Commission appeared to be in favour of the probationer's employee status, there is an interesting recommendation at the end of the section of the Report quoted above (1932b):

Hospitals should recognise that the nurses are paying indirectly, if not directly, for their training, and that the onus rests on the hospitals to provide good facilities for such training, including expert instruction during hours of duty. To this end a ward sister who has to train successive batches of students should be given extra remuneration, and some relief from other duties, for teaching in the wards.

It would seem that this statement, published nearly 40 years ago, has relevance for nursing education today. Students are still paying indirectly for their training and, although ward sisters have been given 'some relief from other duties', the time saved is not necessarily spent in teaching students. Ward sisters in hospitals associated with nursing schools are not required to have had any formal teaching preparation, nor is any extra remuneration paid to ward staff who undertake the teaching of nurses in training.

1.3.3.2 *Changing attitudes towards the employee status of student nurses.* Balme (1937) was one of the first writers to question the student nurse/employee position of nurses in training:

> She is not there as a student, to learn what is the matter with each individual patient and how best to nurse each one. She is there as a piece of ward machinery, to carry out certain duties which have got to be done. They will probably involve doing exactly the same job for each of several patients, but the main criterion by which her work will be appraised is not her understanding of the individual complaints and requirements of each, but the speed with which she can get the work completed.

In her suggestions for experiment in nurse training, Carter (1939) assumes that students in the experimental schemes will be freed from their employee role and will be present in the clinical situation as students. She makes the point on numerous occasions that practice in the ward situation is an essential part of nurse training, but that such practice should be an integral part of a planned and supervised programme.

Since then, a considerable number of reports have been produced on the subject of nurses and nurse training. From these it would appear that an almost continuous crisis situation has existed with regard to the staffing of hospitals.

It is interesting to note that most of the committees and commissions formed by the Government and other interested bodies have concerned themselves with student nurses rather than with trained staff. There is a remarkable similarity between many of these reports. Although there has been some change in attitudes since the Lancet Commission reported, and although there has been a considerable amount of comment on the undesirability of the employee/student situation, the situation itself seems to have been accepted as inevitable. Having commented on the situation, the reports then go on to consider the environmental factors which adversely affect the recruitment and retention of student nurses, and to make recommendations about how the hospital situation can be made more attractive and tolerable—that is, how *working* conditions can be improved so that people will be induced to enter and remain in nursing, without any change being made in their employee/student status.

The Royal College of Nursing (1943), in its *Nursing Reconstruction Committee Report*, said:

> It is obvious that the first essential in the establishment of true nursing education is the

clear separation between the training of nurses and the obligation to provide nursing services for hospital patients.

However, this view was modified a few pages later:

There is nothing incompatible between apprenticeship and studentship, as witness the training of engineers. The nurse trainee must, however, be a student first and an apprentice second... The length of stay in any one department should not depend on the convenience of the hospital.

There would seem to be some dangers in equating engineering and nursing apprentices in this way. The products of the work of the engineering apprentice are more easily subject to inspection and checking than the activities carried out by the nurse apprentice. When the nursing product has been delivered to the patient it is often difficult for the supervising nurse to judge its standard and to return it to the apprentice when adjustment is necessary.

The distinction between studentship and apprenticeship is not always clear. The issue being considered here is the extent to which student nurses are used to provide a service by performing duties which may or may not be necessary or desirable as part of their professional education. The proportion of nursing service provided by students was demonstrated by data collected from a job analysis carried out by the Nuffield Provincial Hospitals Trust (1953c):

Student nurses were found to be, in fact, an indispensable part of the labour force of the wards. Three-quarters of the nursing was contributed by them... Shortages of trained nurses or of domestic workers are compensated by using student nurses.

In the same report an example was given of how a ward sister and a staff nurse spent their time during the peak hours of work between 9 a.m. and 12 noon. The ward sister spent no time at all with students and the staff nurse was in contact with them for only eight minutes.

The Nuffield job analysis was one of the first attempts to study nursing systematically, and to go beyond the collection of opinion, no matter how well informed, offered in evidence to a commission or committee.

1.3.4 Teaching and learning in the clinical situation

1.3.4.1 *Teachers of student nurses.* Throughout her training the student nurse spends periods of time in the classroom where she is taught the theoretical background to nursing, including the biological sciences. The minimum number of lectures to be given in each subject and the qualifications of the lecturers are specified by the General Nursing Council. Lecturers include registered nurse teachers, doctors and, more recently, specialist ward sisters.

However, by far the greater part of the student's time is spent in the clinical situation. What, and by whom, she should be taught in the wards has not been clearly defined.

The three groups of nurses who might be expected to provide most of the ward teaching are ward sisters, staff nurses and clinical instructors. Although they are all registered nurses, only the clinical instructors have had a course of instruction in how to teach. Because there is only a small number of practising clinical instructors, the ward sisters and staff nurses are also expected to teach, in spite of the fact that they lack teaching preparation and are responsible for the total nursing care of the patients.

1.3.4.2 *Ward sisters as teachers.* The teaching role of the ward sister has been the subject of frequent comment. In the *Report of the Working Party on the Recruitment and Training of Nurses* (Ministry of Health *et al* 1947b) it was stated that:

> In a large number of hospitals, formal teaching in the wards is negligible. Many student nurses are taught practically nothing by their ward sisters; others may occasionally pick up odd items of information by sheer chance.

By 1953 there appeared to be a greater awareness of the need for ward teaching. The report by the Nuffield Provincial Hospitals Trust (1953d), *The Work of Nurses in Hospital Wards*, stated that:

> Although the ward sisters and staff nurses were mainly engaged on ward management rather than bedside nursing duties, *the teaching of student nurses did not occupy a prominent place among their duties*, although it was everywhere recognised that it should be so.

Catnach and Houghton (1961) reported that they had great difficulty in assessing the ward teaching which was carried out in a number of schools of nursing in the South-West Metropolitan Area:

> In one hospital, each Ward Sister set aside one hour daily for Ward Reports and discussion of the patients. We were present at two such sessions but nearly all the time was spent on what is admittedly a very important part of the ward routine, namely, the passing on to the nurses coming on duty, details of changes in treatment and instructions about procedures to be carried out. Such information, presumably, would be part of the normal ward routine whether or not student nurses were working in the ward.

It is not quite clear how the authors intended this statement to be interpreted. It could be argued that this time was not spent on teaching. On the other hand, reports of this type could be considered as valuable teaching sessions if they were carefully prepared and presented. The students would then go about their work with up-to-date knowledge of the patients for whom they were providing nursing care.

The report by the Nuffield Provincial Hospitals Trust (1953e) highlights the main points at issue:

> Once the role of the trained nurse is clearly defined and accepted and a satisfactory type of ward organization has been determined in the light of it, the question of the practical training of the student nurse can be seen in its proper perspective. *So long as student nurses comprise more than half the labour force of the wards it is inevitable that their training needs shall be, on occasion, subordinated to administrative necessity.* The only way to ensure that this cannot happen is to evolve a type of ward organization into which they will fit, but which does not *depend* upon them to the present extent. Otherwise, student status will remain a myth.

This does not mean that their training need be entirely theoretical and divorced from that element of practical responsibility which is such an important feature of the tradition of nursing in this country. Placing the responsibility for the student's practical training upon the ward sister is the surest guarantee against this happening. *So long as the minimum nursing care is already provided*, practical work can still be entrusted to student nurses, such work being carried out in conjunction with trained staff and planned in accordance with the student's training.

The work load of ward sisters is a topic of discussion in a number of reports. The Dan Mason Nursing Research Committee (1960a), in its report entitled *The Work, Responsibilities and Status of Staff Nurses*, provided some indications of the amount and pressure of work with which the ward sisters had to cope:

One experienced sister wrote of the pressure of work in her ward of 40 beds which were assigned to five consultants and in addition admitted all female accident cases. She described her day as a series of interruptions divided not into hours or minutes but into seconds.

Another sister who had been in charge of a surgical ward of 28 beds since 1951 stated:

'Each year the rush and speed of work quickens and the [student] nurses have study days depleting our numbers but extra staff is not available. Our patients are rarely able to do much for themselves as they are transferred on the second or third day after operation in order to make room for more patients'.

Under these circumstances, it is hardly surprising that ward sisters have difficulty finding time to teach. In some cases, lack of preparation and experience in teaching may make it difficult for them to utilise the time which is actually available. In spite of this, however, *The Report of the Committee on Senior Nursing Staff Structure* (Ministry of Health, Scottish Home and Health Department, 1966) assumes it to be part of every ward sister's responsibility. 'Teaching of student and pupil nurses' is listed as one of her functions under the suggested job description for the Grade 6, ward sister/charge nurse level of staff.

1.3.4.3 *Staff nurses as teachers.* The staff nurses are the registered nurses with whom students are in closest contact in the wards. When ward sisters are on duty staff nurses are involved in giving direct patient care; if they require assistance it is commonly provided by students. In this situation they would appear to have a contribution to make in teaching students. It may be that they have not been the focus of attention in this context because they have had no formal training as teachers and have had limited opportunity to extend their knowledge of nursing beyond the basic level required for registration.

The position of staff nurses in nursing hierarchy is ill-defined. It would seem that most newly registered nurses spend some time as staff nurses, either as a necessary prerequisite to becoming a ward sister or to fill in time prior to taking further training or getting married.

In the report by The Dan Mason Nursing Research Committee (1956a) on *The Work of Recently Qualified Nurses* it was found that:

Of the *female nurses* who answered, 44.4 per cent were engaged in hospital nursing...

Most of those in hospital practice were staff nurses, some regarded their present posts as temporary, as their future plans indicated, and most of the movement into other branches of nursing was from this group.

The lack of clear definition of the staff nurses' area of responsibility has frequently been the subject of comment. Shortage of staff means that staff nurses may be deputising for ward sisters one day, and doing what they consider to be the work of students, the next. In the above report (1956b) it was said that

...some considered there was insufficient distinction shown between the status of the staff nurse and the nurse in training. Others who had left hospital for district or other nursing appreciated the responsibility and independence of action which was a feature of their present work, preferring it to the subordinate position experienced by them in hospital practice.

In *The Work of Nurses in Hospital Wards* (Nuffield Provincial Hospitals Trust, 1953f), the lack of definition of the staff nurses' responsibilities is dealt with in the following terms:

At present the staff nurse is merely the ward sister's deputy. She has no functional or executive responsibility of her own. There is ample proof that the position is regarded by the nurses themselves simply as a step on the ladder leading to a ward sister's post and most of them do not intend to stay long in it. *It would seem to offer neither the satisfaction of bedside nursing nor executive responsibility.*

Few reports make reference to the staff nurses as teachers of students. The significance placed on this aspect of their work can be deduced from the order in which the staff nurse's responsibilities are presented in the report by The Dan Mason Nursing Research Committee (1960b) on the *Work, Responsibilities and Status of the Staff Nurse:*

The RESPONSIBILITY most frequently mentioned was for nursing treatments which appear to be one of the main occupations of the staff nurse when the sister was busy with administration or ward management. Other items enumerated were responsibility for ordering ward stock, storing and giving drugs and medicines, also supervising and teaching student nurses.

Elsewhere in the same report (1960c), there is evidence to suggest that in the eyes of the ward sisters teaching by staff nurses has relatively low priority. This was indicated in their answers to the question, 'Are the staff nurses' duties so arranged that they can give time to teach and supervise the student nurses?'

Although two-thirds [of the ward sisters] answered yes, the majority explained that teaching and supervision were possible when the staff nurses were working with the student nurses, others qualified their answers by adding 'when time permits'... Only three per cent stated that actual time was allocated for teaching...

This situation would seem to provide staff nurses with intermittent opportunities to improve their nursing skills, but it is doubtful if these make much contribution towards extending their background knowledge of the sciences associated with their work, which includes the teaching of students. Inservice and continuing education for trained staff in hospitals is still very limited and, where facilities are provided, they tend to consist of a few study days each year.

It would seem that the main opportunities to continue their education take three forms: (i) to attend evening classes in their off-duty time, when these are available; (ii) by doing ward rounds with the doctors, during which they are likely to hear discussions about the patients; (iii) private study.

1.3.4.4 *Clinical instructors.* In an effort to make good the deficiencies in the teaching of students in the ward situation, a special six-month course for clinical instructors was instituted by the Royal College of Nursing (Scottish Board) in Edinburgh in 1958. Since then similar courses have been developed in a number of other centres. The General Nursing Council for Scotland recognised the possible advantages of this addition to the teaching staff of the schools of nursing by opening a register for clinical instructors in 1962.

The objectives of introducing clinical instructors were stated by Watkins (1964) to be:

(1) to improve the bedside teaching of the student nurse; (2) to assist the ward sister; (3) to assist the sister tutor.

There have been some problems in relation to the role and status of the clinical instructors (Geddes, 1968), but in spite of these it would seem that this category of nurse teacher has a contribution to make to the practical part of the student nurses' programme.

Unfortunately, many of the advantages which were anticipated did not materialise because there has not been the expected increase in the number of clinical instructors. This may be because they remain on the same salary as that of a ward sister and because there are no promotional prospects for them in schools of nursing.

The idea of having a qualified teacher in the wards, whose primary responsibility is to teach student nurses, is a very attractive one. However, the large number of clinical instructors which would be required to enable them to function effectively makes the proposal somewhat unrealistic. No matter how hard they work, the small number who are at present available makes it impossible for them to visit every ward and teach every student.

Geddes (1968) gives some indication of the numbers which he considers would be required. He suggests that the services of each clinical instructor

...should be restricted to a limited area of the hospital, not more than 60 beds, where she can know both patients and nurses from day to day.

Although it is doubtful whether the number of clinical instructors can usefully be calculated according to the number of beds in areas where students are working rather than according to the number of students, this estimate does draw attention to the quantitative inadequacies of the present situation.

Another limitation associated with the use of clinical instructors, and of particular relevance to the present study, is that they have had little opportunity to extend their knowledge of the scientific background of nursing. Their six-month course of training is geared mainly to teaching them how to pass on the nursing knowledge and skills which they have acquired during their own basic training, and during subsequent professional experience. Their ability to teach the background theory associated with nursing skills is necessarily limited.

It would seem that clinical instructors can, in some situations, make a small contribution to ward teaching, but that their limited number and somewhat restricted educational background are likely to prevent their becoming an important factor in the teaching of nurses in the clinical situation.

1.3.4.5 *Student nurses' views on ward teaching.* When student nurses have been asked their views about the teaching which is provided for them in hospital wards they have indicated that this is a part of nurse training which could be developed and improved. This was the subject of comment in the report of the investigation carried out by the Oxford Area Nurse Training Committee (1966b):

Many students were able to suggest improvements in the training programme. Time and again they suggested more study, more learning and more teaching. They wanted more continuous teaching, more teaching in the ward and greater emphasis on the interrelationship of theory and practice. It is as though the students realised the *potential for teaching* of the situation they are in but feel that so much more could be made of it to the mutual benefit of student and hospital.

It is interesting that Carter (1939) commented:

... most nurses would thankfully give up nine-tenths of their lectures if they could have really efficient teaching on the cases they have to nurse.

In a letter in the *Nursing Times*, Sexton (1970) made the following suggestions for the improvement of nurse training:

That student nurses be removed from the jurisdiction of the hospital authorities and placed under the direct control of the tutorial staff for disciplinary and learning purposes.

Set up twice-yearly revision courses for all trained staff, to keep them in touch with modern day techniques. Also employ ward clerks so that ward sisters can teach...

Treat student nurses as students, this does not mean that they should be divorced from the clinical situation, on the contrary, much of their teaching must take place in the ward as students must receive adequate experience in the care of patients.

Stop using students as the basis of the staff. The D.H.S.S. should educate the general public to appreciate that they are only being nursed by trainees and get them to do something about it.

Night duty should be undertaken by students as experience only. Put the tutors on nights with them.

If nursing students were supernumerary, their theoretical experience could always be related to the ward teaching which would provide the necessary continuity, and save a lot of time.

The views expressed by the writer would appear to represent the opinions of more than one individual since she signed herself in her official capacity as 'Chairman, Rcn Student Section'.

It would seem that student nurses are very aware of the learning opportunities available to them in the wards and also of the potential dangers to the patients which are inherent in the present situation.

1.3.4.6 *Summary of problems of teaching and learning in the clinical situation.* This review of the literature would seem to indicate that all the people involved in clinical teaching and learning are aware of the unsatisfactory nature of the present situation in the wards.

The main points which emerge are:

a. that as long as students remain employees of the Boards of Management, their student role is unlikely to take precedence over their employee role and, because of this, the General Nursing Councils have limited powers of control over how their clinical experience is organised;

b. that the nurses who know most about the patients (ward sisters and staff nurses) do not have (i) the training to enable them to make the best use of teaching opportunities; (ii) an advanced level of knowledge in the biological sciences; (iii) the time to teach;

c. that the clinical instructors who have had teaching preparation, but whose opportunity to advance their knowledge of the biological sciences has been limited, are too few in number to make a meaningful contribution to ward teaching and, as visitors to the wards, they can not know as much about the patients as do the ward sisters and staff nurses;

d. that student nurses are becoming increasingly aware of wasted opportunities for teaching and learning in the wards and are more willing to express their dissatisfaction with the student/employee situation.

1.4 INTELLIGENCE AND SCHOOL ATTAINMENT IN RELATION TO THE EDUCATION OF STUDENT NURSES

1.4.1 Introduction

The knowledge of the biological sciences applied to nursing which the registered nurses have at the end of their training would seem to be acquired in conditions which are not conducive to learning. In these circumstances the students must accept a large part of the responsibility for their own education. The standard of their knowledge will depend to a large extent upon their motivation and their ability to study on their own. Although motivation is important, a proportion of the effectiveness of their studies could be expected to depend upon their level of intelligence, and on their educational experience before entering nursing.

As there is a lack of definition of the standard of knowledge which is required on the completion of nurse training, it is not surprising to find that there is a corresponding lack of information about the levels of intelligence and attainment in school subjects appropriate to entrants to nursing.

1.4.2 Selection of student nurses

The difficulty in identifying suitable candidates may be associated with the fact that the role and functions of nurses practising in different situations have not been identified. For example, the role and functions of registered nurses are different in geriatric wards and in intensive care units; in psychiatric wards and in operating theatres; in hospitals and in the community. It is unlikely, therefore, that there is a 'standard' type of nurse who can function effectively in all situations.

Within the variety of situations in which nurses work a wide variety of abilities are needed. Lancaster (1970), discussing entry standards and recruitment, suggests that:

the range of abilities required in nursing is as wide as the range of patients' needs.

Some provision is already made for meeting the range of needs of patients by having different grades of nursing personnel, but within each grade there is a considerable range of ability.

The Report of the Working Party on Recruitment and Training of Nurses, Ministry of Health *et al.* (1947c), after considering the results of an intelligence test completed by over 2000 nurses, made the comment that:

The extremely wide range of ability in the nursing profession in hospitals shows clearly that it is not to be regarded as a homogeneous group as far as suitability for the profession is concerned. It is inconceivable that persons differing so very widely in their intellectual capacity should respond to the same training or be fitted to discharge the same functions. On the one hand, we have some 40 per cent falling in the top 30 per cent of the population in intelligence; on the other, we have possibly as much as 24 per cent of the profession who are in the lowest 30 per cent of the population in regard to intelligence, and these are not all assistant nurses or pupil assistant nurses... in *absolute* numbers there are more trained and student nurses in hospital at this low level of ability than there are assistant nurses.

Later in the same report (Ministry of Health *et al.*, 1947d) it is recommended that the selection procedure for student nurses should include:

One or more properly standardised tests of intelligence and, if necessary, of scholastic attainments.

So far no great success has been achieved in identifying either the range of intelligence or the level of attainment in school subjects, which is required by candidates suitable for professional nursing preparation. The fact that a high percentage of people who start training abandon it before completion has created interest in the study of the personal characteristics of nurses.

1.4.3 Attrition during nurse training

It is interesting that over the last 30 years there have been only minor changes in the percentages of students who discontinued training. The report just quoted (Ministry of Health *et al.*, 1947e) showed that, between 1940 and 1947,

the wastage of students from general training schools seems to have remained steady... at about 36 to 37 per cent.

The *Annual Report* issued by the General Nursing Council for Scotland, 1970, reveals that between 1965 and 1967 the annual wastage rate was between 32 and 35 per cent.

In the studies which have been done in regard to wastage, the criteria which have been used as measures of success in students have been the completion of the programme and passing the General Nursing Council's registration examinations.

In the main, researchers have tended to concentrate their interest on the people who have withdrawn from nurse training but, as Scott Wright (1968a) points out:

it is not possible to decide if, and to what extent, the students who left differed in some way from those who succeeded in completing the course.

In the study carried out by the Oxford Area Nurse Training Committee (1966c), where the characteristics of stayers and leavers in five schools of nursing were studied, it was found that:

There was no evidence to suggest either that those with certificates were more likely to be successful nor that those with more passes were likely to be more successful than those with a few passes.

On the other hand Scott Wright (1968b), in her study which included 98.5 per cent of student nurses in Scotland in 1961, found that, of the factors studied, those which had the greatest influence on the success of the students were:

the school leaving age, the educational level achieved and the intelligence score of the students...

Later the same report (1968c) goes on to say:

It could indeed be argued... that education was of even greater importance than the intelligence score, but it has to be remembered in this study that only 20 per cent of the students had a school leaving certificate and that the other four fifths of them had to be assessed on the intelligence test alone.*

A good deal of material is available about the many factors which are involved in the recruitment to and the withdrawal of student nurses from training. In 1969, MacGuire reviewed the findings of over 60 research projects. Although she found it difficult to compare the findings in different studies she was able to reach some conclusions about the significance of intelligence levels and school attainment in nurse training:

---

*In 1961 there was no statutory level of education required for entry to schools of nursing.

Exmination success and failure... is not the same thing as overall success in the training programme. Formal educational attainment certificates predict examination success at both the preliminary and final examination stage. Not only are more bright students left to take the final examination but they have a higher pass rate than the survivors from among the less bright entrants...

Because relatively few entrants have formal educational certificates the predictive value of standardized tests is of particular interest. Where these measure intellectual capacity there is a high positive correlation between the test score and success in the preliminary examination. The correlation between test scores and the final examination is not high...

The preliminary and final examinations referred to by MacGuire were those set by the General Nursing Councils for England and Wales and for Scotland.

MacGuire comments on the small number of students who have formal education certificates and the difficulty which this creates in correlating school achievement with criteria of success in nursing.

1.4.4 Educational requirement for entrants to nursing

The opinion has often been expressed that the educational attainment of entrants to nursing should be higher. During the Second World War the entrance qualification and test which were established in 1937 were abandoned and, in spite of efforts made by the General Nursing Council for Scotland, it was not until 1963 that an educational entry requirement was reintroduced in the following form:

... As from the First day of January 1963, no person shall be entitled to commence the training prescribed... for admission to any Part of the Register until she has satisfied the Council that she has passed one of the following educational examinations, namely:

a. a minimum of two passes on the Ordinary Grade of the Scottish Certificate of Education, one of which must be English; or

b. an educational examination of equivalent standard, which is acceptable to the Council; or

c. for an interim period, until a date to be determined by the Council with the consent of the Secretary of State, an educational examination set by the Council.

(Statutory Instruments, 1962)

That many nurse teachers still consider the standard of education for entrants to nursing to be too low was demonstrated by Lancaster (1971) when she asked nurse teachers whether student nurses should be required to have passes at Higher or Advanced level as well as at Ordinary level. The answer 'Yes' was given by 76.4 per cent of the registered nurse teachers, 83.3 per cent of midwife teachers and 76.9 per cent of health visitor tutors.

The statutory educational entry requirements were amended in the *Nurses (Scotland) Rules 1970:*

... (a) a person may enter if she fulfils the following conditions:

... (b) she complies with one of the following educational requirements:

(i) A minimum of two passes on the Ordinary Grade of the Scottish Certificate of education, one of which must be English, and has completed a full-time course of not less than four years in a secondary school or schools, or in a secondary school and an establishment for further education during which time she has studied at least five additional subjects of general education;

(ii) A minimum of three passes on the Ordinary Grade of the Scottish Certificate of Education, one of which must be English;

(iv) Such other educational qualifications as may be acceptable to the Council; or
(v) For an interim period, until a date to be determined by the Council with the consent of the Secretary of State, a pass in an educational examination set by the Council.

(Statutory Instruments, 1970)

It can be seen that there is still a considerable gap between the opinions expressed by the nurse teachers and the new statutory requirements.

As long as the number of students entering nursing with the educational levels of attainment suggested by the nurse teachers remains small, it is difficult to find conclusive evidence to support (or not support) their opinions. Although the General Nursing Councils may decide on what they consider to be the appropriate level of education for entrants to nursing, they do not have the power to change the statutory regulations. Proposed changes must be approved by the Scottish Home and Health Department or the Department of Health and Social Security and inevitably the immediate service needs of the hospitals are taken into consideration rather than the long term effects on nursing service as a whole. More attention is paid to the numbers of students entering nursing than to their abilities and the contribution which they may make to nursing service after completing their training.

1.4.5 The need to study the components of nursing knowledge in relation to measureable abilities (e.g. I.Q. and school attainment)

From this brief review of the literature it can be seen that there is little conclusive evidence as to the optimum levels of intelligence and school attainment which are required by entrants to nursing. Although I.Q. scores and certificates in school subjects have been used in the past to select student nurses, there seems to be only a low or insignificant correlation between these factors and success in the General Nursing Councils' examinations.

However, the studies so far carried out have been concerned with the students' overall success in these examinations. There has been no systematic attempt to analyse the component parts of the knowledge which the examinations are presumably intended to test, and to relate these to any measurable aspect of the nurse's ability. With regard to school attainment, the small percentage of nurses with certificates in school subjects have not provided samples large enough to justify statistical analysis.

In the present study, an attempt will be made to discover the relationship between I.Q. scores and passes in school examination subjects and the component of nursing knowledge which is the subject of this study, that is, the biological sciences.

2. Methods

2.1 INTRODUCTION

The review of studies carried out on nurses and nursing in Britain revealed that no study had been made of the biological sciences related to nursing, and that no methods appropriate to such a study had been developed.

It was decided that the present work should be based on nursing activities currently being carried out by nurses in hospital wards; that nurses' knowledge of the biological sciences relating to these activities should be assessed by means of an objective test (subsequently known as the Science Test); and that doctors should be asked to complete a questionnaire expressing their opinions about the knowledge they assumed nurses to possess in relation to these activities (subsequently known as the Doctors' Questionnaire).

In order to select the nursing activities which were to form the basis of the study it was necessary to find out which nursing activities were carried out in the wards of the hospitals to be included in the study.

A number of informal discussions were held with eight ward sisters to find out if they could provide this information. During these discussions it became clear that they could not be regarded as reliable sources of such information. It was difficult to know whether the varied accounts given by the ward sisters were in fact true accounts of what nurses did in those eight wards, or whether the investigator was being provided with eight opinions of what the ward sisters considered nurses should be doing.

It was, therefore, decided to observe in selected hospital wards and to record (a) the nursing activities which require a knowledge of the biological sciences and (b) how these activities were distributed among the groups of nurses to be studied.

2.2 SAMPLING

2.2.1 Hospitals

The hospitals included in this study were selected with a view to obtaining a wide range of different types of illness and a correspondingly wide range of nursing practices. By doing this it was hoped to reduce the effect of medical specialisation which, because of the specialist interests of the consultants, tends to bring together for treatment in special wards and departments patients suffering from a narrow range of diseases.

Three hospitals were eventually selected:

Hospital 1: a medical teaching hospital with a small proportion of emergency admissions (26 per cent in 1962);

Hospital 2: a small district hospital, not associated with a medical school, which accepted a large proportion of emergency patients (76 per cent in 1962);

Hospital 3: a medical teaching hospital with a large proportion of emergency admissions (48 per cent in 1962).

There was a nursing school attached to each of these hospitals.

Permission to observe in the three hospitals was granted by the Scottish Home and Health Department, the Regional Hospital Board and the Boards of Management of the hospitals. The nursing and medical staff in the hospitals agreed to participate and showed a keen interest in the project.

2.2.2 Wards

The selection of wards for observation was influenced by the availability of male and female units and the degree of medical specialisation. Four wards were used in each of the three hospitals.

In Hospital 1 the two surgical units used for purposes of observation were the only two available. Each ward was in two parts, one for male patients and one for female patients, with 14 and 16 patients respectively. The two medical wards chosen were those with the least specialisation in medical practice. Each had 36 beds situated in a number of rooms and each ward had the same number of male and female patients.

In Hospital 2 there were only three surgical wards; two of these were used, one male and one female. There were only two medical wards, one male and one female. Each of the four wards used had 27 beds.

In Hospital 3 it was possible to observe in one male and one female surgical ward and in one male and one female medical ward, each ward having a different consultant in charge. The surgical wards each had 24 beds and the medical wards 30 beds.

2.2.3 Observation periods

A suitable period of observation in each ward was selected, after consideration of the system of admission of patients in the three hospitals. The aim was that the observer should be present for a period of time sufficient to record the nursing care of patients on emergency admission and thereafter, as well as patients who were admitted from the waiting list for investigation and subsequent treatment.

In one of the hospitals the wards were arranged in pairs, one male and one female ward forming a unit. Each unit was in the charge of a consultant physician or surgeon. Emergency patients were admitted to any one pair of wards throughout a 24 hour period each week. In the other two hospitals emergency patients were admitted, to the selected wards, daily or on alternate days. It was therefore decided to observe and record nursing practices in each ward for a total of seven days. The daytime period consisted of seven consecutive days and the night-time observation was carried out several weeks later on seven consecutive nights. It was felt that by allowing a number of weeks to intervene between the two periods a wider range of nursing practices might be observed, because of the rapid turnover of patients and the variety in the nursing needs of different patient populations.

From Table 1 it will be seen that the average number of days spent by medical and surgical patients in each of the three hospitals was very similar but that medical patients stayed longer than surgical patients.

TABLE 1

AVERAGE LENGTH OF STAY OF PATIENTS
IN THE THREE HOSPITALS

Hospital	Average stay in all medical wards in 1962	Average stay in all surgical wards in 1962
1	20.5 days	13.3 days
2	19.6 days	13.1 days
3	18.8 days	10.9 days

During the daytime observation the observer was present in each ward daily from the time the day staff started in the morning until the night staff started in the evening, except for short breaks at mealtimes. During the night, nursing practices were observed throughout the period of duty of the night nursing staff except for short breaks at mealtimes. Because of the geographical location of the wards and the small number of nurses to be observed, it was possible to record the nursing care given in two wards simultaneously during the night.

The observations in the wards totalled approximately 1800 hours spread over a period of six months.

2.2.4 Nurses

The sample of nurses was drawn from the three hospitals in which nursing activities were observed and consisted of staff nurses, third, second and first year students. Each nurse in the sample agreed to participate in the study after being asked by the investigator if she was willing to do so. The nurses in the sample were not necessarily those who were observed carrying out nursing activities in the wards.

In Hospitals 1 and 2 an attempt was made to include all the nurses of these grades who were on the staff.

In Hospital 1 this aim was not achieved. The main difficulty arose with the staff nurse group as some were on night duty, some on holiday and some of those working in operating theatres found it difficult to be free for the necessary period of time.

TABLE 2

SAMPLE OF NURSES FROM HOSPITAL 1

Group	Total number of nurses	Participants in the study	
		Number	%
Staff nurses	56	42	75.00
3rd year students	73	73	100.00
2nd year students	80	76	95.00
1st year students	72	69	95.83

Most of the nurses in the hospital were given time off from the wards or time during the school day in order to complete the test. No one who was asked actually refused to complete the test but it was not possible to find out if those who could not be free for the necessary period of time offered this reason in preference to saying that they did not wish to participate in the study.

In Hospital 2 the numbers of student nurses and staff nurses were small and an attempt was made to get all the nurses to complete the test. This proved to be impossible because some were on night duty, some on holiday, some on sick leave and a number were on secondment to other hospitals for the specialist clinical experience which was part of their training programme. Only those nurses who were in study blocks in the school of nursing were given time off to complete the tests; the remainder did so in their free time.

TABLE 3

SAMPLE OF NURSES FROM HOSPITAL 2

Group	Total number of nurses	Participants in the study	
		Number	%
Staff nurses	26	18	69.23
3rd year students	15	10	66.67
2nd year students	20	12	60.00
1st year students	24	17	70.83

Hospital 3 had the largest number of staff nurses and student nurses. After consulting a statistician it was decided that if 50 nurses completed the test in each of the four groups, this would provide sample sizes which were statistically acceptable.

It was difficult to gain access to the nurses in this hospital and attempts to select samples of the four groups of nurses by the use of random numbers proved to be impossible for the following reasons:

a. a considerable number of nurses were on night duty, holiday, special and sick leave and on secondment to other hospitals for specialist experience;

b. nurses who had been working in the specialist units in the hospital for some time elected not to participate in the study;

c. nurses were not given time off to complete the test, their off-duty times were frequently changed at short notice and many of those who agreed to participate were unable to keep their appointments.

In the face of these difficulties, the only means by which a sample could be obtained was to accept up to the required number all the nurses who agreed to participate, and who were willing to complete the test in their free time.

The sample of second and third year students consisted of those who were in study blocks in the school of nursing at the time the data were being collected. The students completed the test at the end of the school day. In order to obtain the required numbers of staff nurses and first year students the investigator visited the wards and made appointments for them to complete the test.

All that can be said about the sample from this hospital is that it was stratified according to the four groups of nurses selected to be studied and that the respondents were prepared to go to considerable trouble to participate.

TABLE 4

SAMPLE OF NURSES FROM HOSPITAL 3

Group	Total number of nurses	Participants in the study	
		Number	%
Staff nurses	183	55	30.05
3rd year students	135	53	39.26
2nd year students	152	55	36.18
1st year students	129	52	40.31

TABLE 5

TOTAL SAMPLE OF NURSES FROM THREE HOSPITALS

Hospital	Nurses				
	Staff nurses	3rd year students	2nd year students	1st year students	Total
1	42	73	76	69	260
2	18	10	12	17	57
3	55	53	55	52	215
Total	115	136	143	138	532

It will be seen from Table 4 that the required number of nurses in each group participated in the study and that this was a smaller percentage of the total number in each group than in the other two hospitals. Although the sampling method left much to be desired, the sample sizes were satisfactory for the purposes of statistical analysis.

Table 5 shows the total number of nurses in each group and the hospitals from which they were drawn.

2.2.5 Doctors

Since the doctors who have responsibility for the care of patients in the wards have professional contact with staff nurses, all the doctors in the three hospitals were asked to participate in the study. This produced a total sample of an acceptable size which could be subdivided into the three main grades: consultants, registrars and house officers. A small number of senior house officers were included in the house officer grade.

The medical superintendents of the three hospitals brought the study to the notice of the medical staff, who agreed in principle to participate. It was accepted that each doctor would be free to decide whether he would complete the questionnaire when it was received by him.

It will be seen from Table 6 that 83.64 per cent of the doctors in the three hospitals returned completed questionnaires. Only one doctor in Hospital 1 returned an uncompleted questionnaire. He was a consultant radiologist and indicated that his work did not bring him in contact with staff nurses in relation to the content of the questionnaire. The remaining doctors (34) who did not return the questionnaire gave no reason.

TABLE 6

TOTAL SAMPLE OF DOCTORS FROM THREE HOSPITALS

Hospital	Number of doctors in each hospital	Number who completed the questionnaire	
		Number	%
1	74	58	78.38
2	25	23	92.00
3	115	98	85.22
Total	214	179	83.64

Of the doctors who completed the questionnaire 72 (40.22 per cent) were consultants, 45 (25.14 per cent) were registrars and 62 (34.64 per cent) were house officers.

2.3 DATA COLLECTION

2.3.1 Observation of nursing activities in hospital wards

It was decided to carry out a pilot observation period, consisting of one week of daytime observation, to discover:

a. if it was possible for one observer to record the activities of a number of nurses at the same time;

b. if, with some adjustments, the nursing activities listed in the *Record of Practical Experience* which is provided for student nurses by the General Nursing Council for Scotland could form the basis of a recording schedule to be used in the wards.

A medical ward in Hospital 1 was chosen for the pilot observation because immediate access was available. As the patients occupied a number of rooms, it was felt that it might be difficult to observe several nurses at the same time. If it proved possible in this ward, it would be easier in the other selected wards.

The list of nursing activities taken from the official *Record of Practical Experience* was found to be inadequate as an observation guide because many nursing practices were not performed in their entirety by one nurse. On some occasions one nurse prepared the equipment and the patient for the treatment, but was called away to attend to the immediate needs of another patient and the treatment was completed by another nurse; on some occasions subsequent adjustments to the apparatus were made by a third nurse. This situation created recording problems when the second and possibly the third nurse involved were not in the same year of training as the first. One example of how the list had to be adjusted may be cited.

The *Record of Practical Experience* has an entry: 'Administration of Oxygen'. In the first week of observation, this single item had to be expanded into:

Administration by B.L.B. mask	preparation for setting up apparatus
Administration by polymask	preparation for setting up apparatus
Administration by oxygen tent	preparation for setting up apparatus
Administration by venturi apparatus	preparation for setting up apparatus

Adjustment of the supply of oxygen.

The first week of observation showed that it was possible for one observer to record the activities of several nurses, some of them students and some of them staff nurses. This was possible because the observer made no attempt to evaluate the nursing care given, or to remain with the nurse throughout the time taken to carry out the treatment. The observer simply recorded that a nurse was preparing for or carrying out a treatment and, while this treatment was being done, checked whether all other nurses were continuing with what they were last seen to be doing or were changing to some other activity. A knowledge of nursing practice was of considerable value, as the observer was able to estimate the length of time which the nurses would take to prepare for, or to perform, an item of nursing care.

Adjustments were made to the list of nursing activities until a satisfactory recording schedule had been constructed.

The Boards of Management of the hospitals concerned in the study agreed that photographs could be taken in the wards during the observation period. It was intended that these photographs should be representative of the nursing practices observed, and that they be shown to student nurses and staff nurses as an orientation to the nursing practices about which questions would be asked later, when the Science Test was administered.

During the initial period of observation, an Ilford black and while film in a 35 mm f2.8 Minolta Uniomat camera with built in rangefinder and uncoupled exposure meter was used. The assessment of suitable exposure was found to be difficult because of the position of beds in the wards. Beds are commonly situated with the head against an outside wall with a window on each side. Most photographs had to be taken towards the head of the bed, and thus towards a darker area flanked by two brighter areas. End prints were taken from the first roll of film exposed but, on the whole, they were unsatisfactory. It was decided at this time that the most suitable method of presenting the photographs to nurses completing the Science Test would be by projected transparencies. All subsequent photographs were taken on coloured Perutz film using electronic flash to overcome lighting difficulties. In this way, satisfactory transparencies were obtained during both day and night-time observation. The photographs were taken of nursing situations as they existed in the wards. Artificial situations were not created for this purpose. Some photographs were taken in each hospital and wherever possible a nurse was included in the scene. It was felt that the slides would provide a more effective orientation to the test questions if the ward and the nurse in the uniform of the hospital were recognised. Before they were used the slides were treated to ensure that the patients could not be identified.

2.3.2 Selection of nursing activities from observations in hospital wards

The total number of items on the list which was used to record nursing activities in the wards was 172. This large number was the result of having to fragment each activity in order to record accurately which nurses had been involved in it. The separate parts of the nursing procedure carried out by different nurses had to be recorded as separate observations. This detailed type of recording was also necessary when a treatment was continued for a relatively long period of time. For example, bladder irrigation and drainage was subdivided as follows:

Item observed	Frequency
Collection and assembly of the equipment	11
Setting up the apparatus	11
Changing bottles of irrigating fluid	41
Adjusting the rate of flow of fluid	65
Total	128

The different parts of an activity were summed and the total figure used to convey how frequently the activity was observed. This reduced the list to 75 nursing practices. As the list still contained too many items for a question to be included on each, it was decided to group the items on the basis of the overlap in their science content. Finally, a list was derived of 22 activities which subsumed the 75 in the condensed list described above.

The following is an example of the grouping of activities carried out.

The heading 'Administration of drugs' included administration by different routes: oral, rectal or by injection. These items are all concerned with the administration of drugs as a whole, and the associated question concerned drugs in general. All of these activities require an understanding of the measurement of doses of drugs and this aspect was included in another question. Giving drugs by injection involves an understanding of the principles of sterilisation of equipment and the use of aseptic technique, both of which were included in other questions.

2.3.3 Nurses' Science Test

Twenty-two questions were prepared for presentation to the nurses. Each question was based on a nursing activity which had been observed in the wards, and which would be recognised as a commonly occurring nursing practice by the nurses completing the test.

The questions included scientific principles applicable to a number of different nursing practices. Each principle was 'attached' to a particular activity, for example, principles underlying the use of aseptic techniques were 'attached' to a question about doing a surgical dressing. These principles applied to many other activities during which a patient could be at risk by the introduction of pathogenic micro-organisms through the skin, through the mucous membrane or into the urinary system. Activities in this group include giving injections, dressing wounds, passing a catheter into the bladder, preparing for activities performed by a doctor, such as the aspiration of fluid from body cavities or the withdrawal of blood from a vein.

The questions formulated were of the 'objective' type. These were in two forms; matching and multiple choice questions.

a. In the matching type of question a number of details of the method of the procedure were listed in one column and at least twice as many 'reasons' for the use of these accepted practices were provided in a second column. The nurses were asked to 'pair off' the appropriate detail of practice with the 'true' reason for its use. In the second column there was only one 'true' reason for each item of technique. The question formulated on aseptic technique, which was discussed earlier, provides an example of this type of question:

Surgical dressings are commonly performed by nurses. Column A consists of a number of important points of aseptic technique and some of the items in column B the reasons for them. Place the number of the item in column A beside the appropriate reason in Column B.

No.	Column A	Column B	Place correct no. here
1.	The nurse doing the dressing washes and dries her hands carefully	To prevent contamination of the atmosphere	
2.	The soiled dressing is removed with forceps used for that purpose only	Prevents atmospheric contamination of the depths of the wound	
3.	Drainage from a wound should be into a closed receptacle	The organisms may be antibiotic resistant	
4.	When a stitch is being removed it should be cut very close to the skin surface	Micro-organisms spread quickly in a moist medium	
5.	A dry dressing is preferred to a lotion dressing	Prevents the spread of micro-organisms to the new dressing	
6.	Sterile instruments should be used to handle dressings	To develop manual dexterity	
		Antiseptics inhibit the growth of organisms	
		To avoid introducing bacteria from the skin into the deeper layers of tissue	
		Disinfectants kill organisms but damage healthy tissue	
		When many dressings are being done the skin of the hands may become cracked	
		A wound can seal itself from possible infection only when it is dry	
		Instruments can be sterilised but hands can be regarded as sterile only when sterile gloves are worn	

b. In the multiple choice questions nurses were asked to select the correct items from at least twice as many choices as there were correct items. The question on the factors which influence the blood concentration of a drug provides an example of this type:

A specific blood concentration of a drug must be maintained in order to provide effective treatment of the condition from which the patient is suffering. Place a tick beside those factors in the following list which affect the blood concentration of the drug.

Please tick here

1. The rate of absorption from the alimentary tract
2. The toxicity of the drug
3. The size of the patient
4. The volume of urine excreted
5. The amount of exercise taken by the patient
6. The frequency of dosage
7. The fact that the drug acts selectively on some tissues and not on others
8. The solubility of the drug in the body fluids
9. The rate of excretion of the drug
10. The ability of the liver to destroy the drug

In the nurses' test as it was used initially there were 14 matching and eight multiple choice questions. The test in its final form, which contained 19 questions, had 12 matching and seven multiple choice questions.

When the test was scored no corrections to the nurses' scores were made to compensate for guessing. Vernon (1956a) points out that:

...the examinee's shaky knowledge may not always be to his advantage. For the alternative (wrong) answers are usually worded sufficiently plausibly to deceive the weak student, and should indeed be based on common misconceptions. Hence his 'semi-guesses' will in practice be very frequently wrong.

Vernon goes on later to explain that such corrections may, indeed, over-compensate for guessing. He also discusses the relationship between the time allowed for the test and guessing:

...correction becomes less necessary the longer the time allowance for the examination. (Vernon, 1956b)

Both of these ideas were taken into account when formulating the questions and administering the test. Common misconceptions were used in making up the wrong answers which were offered and no time limit for the completion of the Science Test was imposed.

After the Science Test was prepared it was submitted for scrutiny to other members of the staff of the Nursing Studies Unit of the University of Edinburgh and to the group of students who were in the second year of their two year preparation as nurse teachers, having completed a course on biological sciences in the first year. They were asked to answer four questions:

a. Could they understand the preamble to each question?

b. Did they consider the question items to be appropriate to the nursing activity represented?

c. Did they agree with the correct answers to the questions?

d. Did they consider the alternative answers offered to be wrong but representative of common misconceptions?

Some adjustments were made to the questions as a result of the comments provided.

The Science Test was then presented to a group of 30 nurses in Hospital 1 to find out if there were any questions which were not understood. This hospital was used for the preliminary use of the Science Test because of the easy access to the nurses which was made possible by the nursing administration and tutorial staffs.

The results showed that there was no question which was incomprehensible to the whole group. It was decided, however, to remove three questions which asked for information about how specific activities should be carried out; these questions did not adequately test the nurses' knowledge of the biological sciences upon which the activities depend. As some of the nurses expressed the view that the test was too long (it took about 75 minutes), it was decided that two purposes could be served by the removal of these three questions.

In its final form the Science Test contained 19 questions. The scores obtained on these questions by the 30 nurses who attended the preliminary session were included in the main study.

Nursing education is generally considered to be progressive throughout the three years. If this applied to nursing practice in the wards then it could be expected that less complex tasks would be carried out by the more junior students and the more complex tasks carried out by senior students and staff nurses. There was little evidence of this type of grading of activities during the period of observation in the wards.

Because of this no attempt was made to grade the questions in terms of difficulty. The same questions were used for all groups of nurses. On the other hand no attempt was made to standardise the questions so that they would all be equally difficult. This did not appear to be necessary because the scores of which group of nurses, on each question and on the Science Test as a whole, were to be compared with each other, and the staff nurses' scores were to be compared with the doctors' expectations of their knowledge. The test scores were not to be graded according to any arbitrary pass/fail standard.

2.3.4 Nurses' intelligence (I.Q.) and school attainment

Many of the reports published about nurses and nursing education included comment on the levels of intelligence and of attainment in school subjects of entrants to the profession. Student nurses and staff nurses were therefore asked to complete an intelligence test and to provide information about the passes they had gained in school subjects so that these could be correlated with their scores in the Science Test.

One of the hospital schools had for a number of years used the Otis Self-Administering Test of Mental Ability, Intermediate Examination, as part of its methods of selecting student nurses. As these results were available, and the respondents agreed to their use, the same test was given to the nurse respondents in the other two hospitals. Some of the staff nurses in the first hospital who were not trainees of the nursing school also agreed to do the test.

Two forms of the Otis Self-Administering Test are available; the Intermediate and Higher Examinations. For students entering schools of nursing, the Higher Examination might have been more appropriate but, as indicated above, the Intermediate Examination was already in use in one of the schools of nursing.

As explained by Otis (a) in the *Manual of Directions and Key*:

The Intermediate Examination is designed for senior schools and the middle forms of secondary schools.

Although this is a younger age group than the sample of nurses included in the present study, norms are provided for eighteen years of age and over. The examination consists of 75 items and the norm for this age group is 59 (I.Q. = 100).

The *Manual* does not give the actual numbers of school pupils upon whom the norms for the Intermediate Examination are based but Super and Crites (1960) state that:

The age and grade norms are based on large samples from various sections of the United States, neither a random nor a stratified sample, but one large and varied enough so that to assume its adequacy seems sound...

In the *Manual of Directions and Key* Otis (b) explains that the tests were standardised by using the scores obtained from 1000 high school and 1000 grammar school pupils in different parts of the United States:

...the students were divided... into two groups, a 'good group' and a 'poor group'. The same number were taken from each grade for both groups. The good group constituted the young students, and the poor group the old students. These groups had reached the same average educational status, therefore, but at different rates. Now it is the rate at which a student can progress through school that the mental-ability test is chiefly used to predict... Each item justified its inclusion, therefore, because it distinguished between students who progressed slowly and those who progressed rapidly.

Super and Crites (1960b) pointed out that:

Strictly adult norms have not been published, despite widespread use at that age level.

The same writers also point out that the standardisation method was of an academic type and that these tests may not be particularly good predictors of performance in non-academic occupations. Correlates between the Otis test and a variety of aspects of some occupations are available. Relationships between success in the examination of the General Nursing Council for Scotland and the Otis Intermediate Test are reported by Scott Wright (1961), but these results are not comparable with the findings of the present study which is confined to biological sciences related to nursing.

2.3.5 Presentation of the Science and Intelligence Tests to the nurses

It was decided that the Science Test should be completed in the presence of the investigator as freedom to consult textbooks would defeat the purpose of the test.

Classroom conditions, including the use of a slide projector and a screen, were required for the administration of the Science Test. When a classroom in the hospital school of nursing was not available, sessions were held in the Nursing Studies Unit. The hospital school facilities were used wherever possible as these were more convenient for the nurses.

When intelligence test scores were not already available the two tests were completed at the same session.

The number of nurses who were present at the different sessions varied from three to 45.

A pattern of presentation of the tests was established at the first session and was maintained throughout. When the group had assembled the explanation of the study which they were given when they were asked to participate was repeated, and questions were invited and answered. The intelligence test was timed to take 30 minutes and was presented first, using the standard instructions provided. This was followed by showing the orientation transparencies and as each was shown the nursing activity which it represented was named. Before the Science Test was handed out, the nurses were told that they had unlimited time in which to answer the questions and could leave when they had finished.

Sessions of a similar pattern were repeated until the total sample of 532 nurses had been tested.

2.3.6 Doctors' questionnaire

The questions which were formulated for presentation to doctors were based on the same nursing activities as those which provided the basis of the nurses' Science Test.

Three types of question were asked:

Group A (questions 1-7)

These questions were subdivided into the same items as were the nurses' questions. The doctors were provided with the items and the answers, and were asked if they considered that a staff nurse should have this knowledge. An example of this type of question is given below.

Surgical dressings are treatments commonly performed or supervised by the staff nurse. Place a tick beside those items with which you consider the staff nurse should be familiar, without specific prescription, if she is responsible for this work.

Please
tick here

1. The nurse doing the dressing washes and dries her hands to prevent the easy spread of organisms in a moist medium

2. That soiled dressings are removed with forceps used for that purpose only in order to prevent the contamination of the new dressing

3. That drainage of a wound should be into a closed receptacle to prevent contamination of the depths of the wound

4. When a stitch is being removed it is cut very close to the skin to prevent the introduction of bacteria from the skin into the deeper layers of tissue

5. That a dry dressing and access to the air is preferred to a moist closed dressing to encourage the wound to seal itself

6. That sterile instruments should be used to handle dressings and not the hands as the hands can never be considered as sterile unless sterile gloves are worn

Group B (questions 8-11)

These questions were subdivided into the same items as were the nurses' questions but the answers were not given. The doctors were asked whether they would prescribe in such detail and if they would expect the staff nurses to initiate items of activity. An example of this type of question is given below:

Place a tick beside the items of preventive care of pressure areas in the following list which you consider the staff nurse should initiate without specific prescription.

                                                                           Place
                                                                         tick here

1. Frequent change of position of the patient

2. Changing linen, washing and drying of the area if it is contaminated if the patient is incontinent

3. Early ambulation if there are no contraindications

4. Special attention to the diet especially the protein and vitamin content

5. The use of air rings, wool rings, slings and pulleys if the patient must remain in one position

Group C (questions 12-19)

This group consisted of those questions in which there was not direct comparability between the doctors' responses and the staff nurses' scores. In these questions doctors were asked if they would expect staff nurses to initiate and take responsibility for specific activities associated with patient care. An example of this type of question is given below:

Some drugs may be prescribed in metric measure and dispensed in imperial measure or vice versa. If such a drug is prescribed would you consider it the responsibility of the staff nurse in charge of the ward to ensure that the patient received the dose?

1. Always

2. Sometimes

3. Never

In interpreting the doctors' answers to the questions it was assumed that the doctors expected the staff nurses to have a detailed knowledge of an activity if they indicated that:

a. they would not prescribe the details enumerated in the question or
b. they assumed that the staff nurses would initiate and take responsibility for the activity as a whole.

2.3.7 Presentation of the Questionnaire to the doctors

On the advice of the medical superintendents of the three hospitals the questionnaires were sent out by mail immediately after the doctors had been reminded of the study at a medical staff meeting.

An explanatory letter and a stamped addressed envelope were included with the questionnaire.

In response to this initial request 162 questionnaires were returned within two weeks. A second letter and copy of the questionnaire were sent to the non-respondents after two weeks which resulted in a further 17 questionnaires being returned completed. The final number of non-respondents was 35 (see Table 6).

2.4 STATISTICAL ANALYSIS OF DATA

The data upon which analyses were carried out were obtained from the observations of activities carried out in the wards, the nurses' Science Test and the Doctors' Questionnaire.

a. The frequency of observations of each activity carried out in the wards by each group of nurses was expressed as a percentage of the total number of times the activity was seen to be carried out. Percentages were used because the total frequency of observation of each activity was different.

b. For the nurses in each group scores were obtained on the Science Test as a whole, on the individual questions, on the items within each question, and on the intelligence test. Personal information was obtained from each nurse about the number of passes attained in school subjects before entering nursing.

c. From the Doctors' Questionnaire the number of responses to each question and to each item in the questions was obtained. Each doctor provided information about his grade in the National Health Service, that is, consultant, registrar or house officer. Senior house officers were few in number and were included with house officers.

Analysis of variance was used to test the significance of the differences between: (i) mean scores of groups of nurses; (ii) the mean scores of nurses and the mean expectations of doctors; (iii) the mean expectations of the different grades of doctor; and (iv) mean doctors' expectations as elicited by the three types of question.

There were two reasons for using this method to test the significance of the differences between means. Firstly a one-tailed test was appropriate because it was hoped that information could be obtained from the data as to whether one group of respondents had 'superior' knowledge (or expectations) and not merely that a difference existed between the samples (Lewis, 1967). Secondly, the proportion of total variance can be attributed to that part which is within the component distributions and that which is between the means of the combined distributions (Garrett, 1958a).

It was expected, before the data were collected, that staff nurses would have superior knowledge of the biological sciences as compared with student nurses, and that with each year of seniority student nurses would have acquired more knowledge. Also, it was expected that the doctors would assume that the staff nurses had more knowledge of these sciences than they did in fact display.

In relation to the assumptions of the staff nurses' knowledge expressed by the different grades of doctor, it was expected that the more senior the grade of doctor the greater would be their assumptions of the staff nurses' knowledge. In relation to the types of question used in the Doctors' Questionnaire it was expected that in those questions where less detailed information was given about the scientific knowledge involved, the doctors' assumptions of the staff nurses' knowledge would be demonstrably greater.

In the Group C questions, which required an 'always/sometimes/never' answer, the response of the three grades of doctor were tested by the chi-square test to find if the differences between the grades were significant. This test was also used when comparing the scores of the different groups of nurses in question 16 in the Science Test in which there was only one right answer. The standard deviation was calculated using the total scores of the nurses in each group. For this purpose the Short Method described by Garrett (1958b) was applied directly to the ungrouped scores.

In calculating the coefficient of correlation between the scores of the four groups of nurses and the frequency with which each was observed to carry out activities associated with the questions asked in the Science Test, Spearman's rank-difference method was used (Garrett, 1958 c). It was felt that ranking the scores and the frequencies of observation was the most appropriate method of finding out if the groups who had most knowledge of the biological sciences upon which an activity is based were the groups who carried out the activity most frequently, and vice versa. For this purpose scores and frequencies of observation of activities were expressed as percentages. The ranking of the frequencies of observation of activities as raw data would have been distorted by the differences in total frequencies with which individual activities were observed.

Coefficients of correlation were calculated between the scores in the Science Test of the nurses in each group and (i) their I.Qs. and (ii) their attainment in school subjects. These were calculated by using Pearson's product-moment method where raw scores and their deviations from zero were used (Garrett, 1958d).

2.5 DEFINITION OF TERMS

Staff nurses (N = 115): respondents who were registered general nurses.

3rd Year students (N = 136): nurses who had completed two years of training but had not yet sat the final examination of the General Nursing Council.

2nd Year students (N = 143): nurses who had completed the Preliminary State Examination and were in their second year of training.

1st Year students (N = 138): nurses who had not yet sat the Preliminary State Examination.

Doctors (N = 179): the total sample of doctors who completed the questionnaire. Where the sample was divided into three levels of seniority this was done according to the positions which the doctors held in the medical staffing structure of hospitals: *consultants* (N = 72), *registrars* (N = 45) and *house officers* (N = 62).

Science Test: an objective test containing nineteen questions on the biological sciences applied to nursing, presented to a sample of 532 registered and student nurses.

Doctors' Questionnaire: a questionnaire based on the same nursing activities as those in the nurses' Science Test, presented to 179 doctors. They were asked to state: (i) whether they would expect staff nurses to have the knowledge specified in the questions (Group A and B questions), (ii) whether they would expect staff nurses to initiate and take responsibility for some nursing procedures (Group C questions).

Doctors' expectations: the doctors' responses to the questions and items in the Doctors' Questionnaire.

Activities: nineteen nursing practices each of which provided the basis for a question in the nurses' Science Test and the Doctors' Questionnaire.

For the sake of convenience, shortened titles have been used to indicate the activity involved in each question. Similar titles are used in the text and the tables. Because of their brevity they are not intended to describe the content of the questions.

Items: the component parts of an activity. The questions in the nurses' Science Test and in Group A and B questions in the Doctors' Questionnaire were made up of a number of items.

Significance of difference between staff nurses' scores and doctors' 'expectations' and between the scores of different groups of nurses: differences are described as *highly significant* if the probability of this difference occurring by chance is less than 0.01 ($p < .01$) and *significant* if the probability is between 0.05 and 0.01 ($p < .05$). If the probability of a difference occurring by chance is greater than 0.05 ($p > 0.5$) it is considered that there is *no significant difference*.

3. Findings: Staff Nurses and Doctors

3.1 INTRODUCTION

It was indicated in the introduction that the staff nurses' knowledge of the biological sciences associated with certain nursing activities would be compared with the doctors' responses to questions based on the same activities, and that the doctors' responses would be used as an indication of the standard of knowledge of the biological sciences appropriate to the practising registered nurse.

The data from the nurses' Science Test and the Doctors' Questionnaire will be presented in the following parts:

(a) Comparison of the staff nurses' scores and the doctors' expectations of the staff nurses' knowledge in Group A and B questions (1-11). In the Doctors' Questionnaire these questions were broken down into items which were comparable with those in the questions presented to staff nurses.

(b) Discussion of the staff nurses' scores and of the doctors' expectations in relation to Group C questions (12-19). In the Doctors' Questionnaire these questions were not statistically comparable with those in the staff nurses' Science Test. They were stated in more general terms, asking doctors if they would expect staff nurses to initiate and take responsibility for certain nursing activities.

(c) Comparison of the staff nurses' scores and the doctors' expectations of the staff nurses' knowledge of the items in Group A and B questions (1-11) classified according to the different biological sciences.

(d) Comparison of the doctors' expectations of the staff nurses' knowledge in all the questions according to the grade of doctor: consultants, registrars and house officers.

(e) Comparison of the doctors' responses according to the three types of question.

3.2 COMPARISON OF STAFF NURSES' SCORES IN THE SCIENCE TEST WITH DOCTORS' EXPECTATIONS OF THE STAFF NURSES' KNOWLEDGE

3.2.1 Comparison of staff nurses' scores in questions in Science Test with doctors' expectations of the staff nurses' knowledge

3.2.1.1 *Group A and B questions: 1 to 11* (Table 7, p. 55). In these groups of questions the content was the same in the staff nurses' Science

Test and in the Doctors' Questionnaire. For each question the staff nurses' knowledge were compared by analysis of variance (Garrett, 1958a). Details of the figures used for this analysis are in Table 7, p. 55.

It was found that in only one question there was no significant difference between the means. In the remaining ten questions the differences between means were highly significant. In eight of these the mean doctors' expectations was higher than the mean staff nurses' score, and in two the mean staff nurses' score was higher than the mean doctors' expectations.

Question 6 was the only one where there was no significant difference between the mean staff nurses' score and the mean doctors' expectations. The subject of this question was disinfection of the bath.

Early ambulation of patients has meant that more patients use the bath more frequently during their stay in the wards. It was noticed during the period of observation in the wards that bathing in the bath was prescribed for some patients as treatment to assist wound healing. Some of these patients had wound infections.

During the period of observation patients were seen to be bathed in the bath 367 times, mainly between 10 a.m. and 12.30 p.m., and in each ward only one bath was available. Disinfection of the bath was therefore of considerable importance in the prevention of cross infection.

The two questions in which the staff nurses' mean score was higher than the mean doctors' expectations were on the subjects of preparing the patient for operation (question 4) and on weighing patients in the wards (question 11).

In the question on the preparation of patients for operation there were six items; the staff nurses' mean score was 5.70 and the mean doctors' expectations was 4.22.

The lower mean doctors' expectations may be the result of physicians having ideas different from those of the surgeons about the preparation of the patient for operation. However, as only 10 (5.6 per cent) of the doctors did not answer the question, the majority of the physicians indicated that they had an opinion to express.

In the question on weighing patients in the wards there were six items. The mean staff nurses' score was 4.30; the mean doctors' expectations 3.45. The staff nurses were asked to select the circumstances under which weighing of patients is common practice, and the doctors were asked if they would expect the staff nurses to initiate weighing of patients under the same circumstances.

There was a somewhat high 'no response' to this question. Twenty-nine (16.2 per cent) doctors indicated that they would not expect the staff nurses to initiate weighing of the patients in any of the situations presented in the question.

In the remaining eight questions, that is, in 72.7 per cent of the questions, the doctors' expectations of the staff nurses' knowledge were higher than the staff nurses' scores.

FIGURE 1 (SEE TABLE 7)

STAFF NURSES' SCORES IN SCIENCE TEST AND DOCTORS'
EXPECTATIONS OF STAFF NURSES' KNOWLEDGE

Comparison of means in questions where the difference was significant

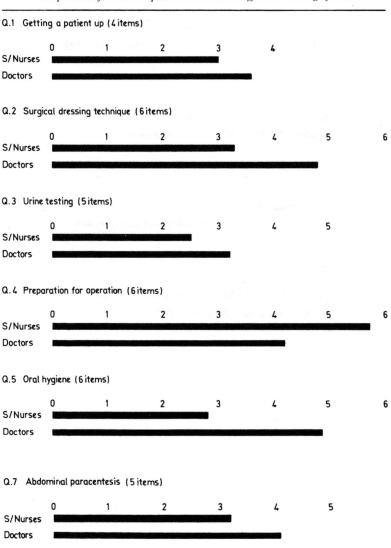

FIGURE 1 CONTINUED (SEE TABLE 7)

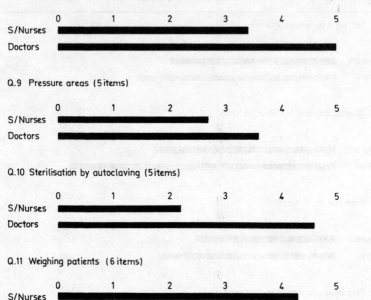

Q.8   Collection of specimens: microbiological (6 items)

Q.9   Pressure areas (5 items)

Q.10 Sterilisation by autoclaving (5 items)

Q.11 Weighing patients (6 items)

TABLE 7

STAFF NURSES' SCORES IN SCIENCE TEST AND DOCTORS' EXPECTATIONS OF THE STAFF NURSES' KNOWLEDGE (GROUP A and B QUESTIONS)

Question number, activity, respondents	Staff nurses' scores (N = 115) Doctors' expectations (N = 179) Number of items:							Totals	Means	Significant differences df = 293 F - ratio
	0	1	2	3	4	5	6			
1. *Getting a patient up*										
Staff nurses	5	5	24	37	44	-	-	340	2.96	29.28
Doctors	3	4	13	27	132	-	-	639	3.57	$P < .01$
2. *Surgical dressing technique*										
Staff nurses	2	9	16	40	27	16	5	379	3.30	63.93
Doctors	16	0	1	9	18	49	86	862	4.82	$P < .01$
3. *Urine testing*										
Staff nurses	2	26	31	35	16	5	-	282	2.45	15.51
Doctors	25	16	14	33	25	66	-	573	3.20	$P < .01$
4. *Preparation for operation*										
Staff nurses	0	1	2	2	1	13	96	656	5.70	440.12
Doctors	10	6	14	25	29	39	56	756	4.22	$P < .01$
5. *Oral hygiene*										
Staff nurses	8	10	31	28	25	9	4	325	2.82	141.76
Doctors	3	4	11	13	16	40	92	881	4.92	$P < .01$
6. *Bathing patient: disinfection of bath*										
Staff nurses	1	6	21	32	35	20	-	384	3.34	1.09
Doctors	9	15	28	26	24	77	-	630	3.52	
7. *Abdominal paracentesis*										
Staff nurses	3	9	12	40	35	16	-	373	3.24	40.78
Doctors	2	6	7	30	39	95	-	741	4.14	$P < .01$
8. *Collection of specimens: (microbiological)*										
Staff nurses	2	8	24	23	27	24	7	395	3.43	110.53
Doctors	0	1	4	11	35	60	68	890	4.97	$P < .01$
9. *Pressure areas*										
Staff nurses	4	9	41	32	17	12	-	315	2.74	39.33
Doctors	1	0	24	63	56	35	-	636	3.55	$P < .01$
10. *Sterilisation by autoclaving*										
Staff nurses	13	16	35	36	14	1	-	255	2.22	249.29
Doctors	11	1	0	4	6	157	-	822	4.59	$P < .01$
11. *Weighing patients*										
Staff nurses	2	0	5	15	40	39	14	494	4.30	15.17
Doctors	29	9	22	24	27	23	45	618	3.45	$P < .01$

3.2.1.2 *Group C questions: 12 to 19* (Table 8, p. 60). In this group of questions the doctors were asked about their expectations of action which might be taken by the staff nurses in association with specific activities and situations. With the exception of question 12, they were not asked what knowledge they would expect the staff nurse to have in order to take such action.

As in Group A and B questions, the staff nurses were asked itemised questions in order to elicit their background knowledge of the biological sciences involved in the activity or situation.

No statistical analysis was done using the data from Group C questions as the staff nurses' scores and the doctors' responses were not directly comparable.

In question 12 the staff nurses were asked to select physiological factors associated with the maintenance of the normal blood pressure. The doctors were asked to indicate their expectations of the staff nurses' knowledge of some pathological changes which affect the factors associated with the maintenance of blood pressure. The staff nurses' score and the doctors' expectations could not be compared because the doctors' question did not discriminate between physiology and pathology. On the physiology, the staff nurses' score was 70.1 per cent, and on the combined pathology and physiology the doctors' expectations of the staff nurses' knowledge was 58.9 per cent of the items included in the question.

Question 17 dealt with one of the most commonly prescribed treatments for patients in hospital, the administration of drugs. During the period of observation 6568 doses were seen to be administered. In prescribing the dose and the frequency with which it has to be given, the doctor is concerned to maintain the blood concentration of the drug at a therapeutic level. There are occasions on which the patient cannot be given the dose at the prescribed time, and sometimes the patient vomits immediately after the dose has been given. The doctors were asked to indicate, through the examples provided, when they would expect the staff nurses to take the initiative in restoring the therapeutic blood level of the drug. The staff nurses were asked to select, from a list of factors, those which would affect the blood concentration of a drug.

The staff nurses' score on this question was 76.2 per cent, and the doctors' expectations 60.3 per cent. Although the doctors' expectations are expressed as a percentage, it must be appreciated that this is a percentage of the possible number of responses offered in the question and cannot be assumed to include all the situations in which the doctors would expect staff nurses to take this type of action.

This result suggests that doctors do expect nurses to use their judgment in order to achieve the aims of prescribed medical treatment. The doctors' responses to this question are indicative of the considerable understanding which exists between doctors and nurses in the working situation. It is probably that arrangements made verbally between doctors and registered nurses are effective in ensuring that the objectives of prescribed treatments are achieved.

Question 16 was about the regulation of intravenous infusion which was observed in the wards 769 times. The staff nurses were asked to indicate the rate of flow which would be necessary in order that 500 ml of fluid could be given in 4 hours. The doctors were asked how they would prescribe the patients' intravenous infusion. During the period of observation a variety of methods of prescribing were observed, none of which included the rate of flow in drops per minute. If the doctors did not prescribe in drops per minute and the nursing staff were expected to organise the flow of fluid, it would seem that the doctors assumed that the nurses had the relevant knowledge.

Only 3 doctors (1.7 per cent) said that they would include the rate of flow in drops per minute in their prescription and only 16.5 per cent of the staff nurses gave the correct answer to the mathematical problem. It could be argued that staff nurses know from experience when the rate of flow 'looks right', but it would seem to be a somewhat hazardous situation for the patient while they are acquiring this experience.

In the remaining five questions the doctors were asked whether they would expect the staff nurses to initiate and take responsibility for activities which may or may not have been prescribed. The questions were formulated in general terms, and the doctors were provided with a three-point scale on which to reply: always, sometimes, never.

The staff nurses were asked itemised questions to elicit their knowledge of the sciences upon which each of the activities is based.

In Figure 4 the staff nurses' scores in these questions are included for interest only as no statistical comparisons were made.

In question 13 the doctors were asked if they would expect the staff nurses to set up prescribed bladder irrigation and drainage for a patient after prostatectomy, when they were absent from the ward. The 24 per cent 'no reply' to this question is probably accounted for by the fact that this activity is not encountered by physicians. Of the doctors who replied, 65.9 per cent said they would always expect the staff nurses to carry out this activity.

The staff nurses' score on this question was 56.5 per cent.

In question 14, on the subject of sterilisation of equipment by boiling, 84.4 per cent of the doctors said they would always expect the staff nurses to take the responsibility for this activity. Only 1.7 per cent of the doctors gave no reply.

The staff nurses' score on this question was 52.9 per cent.

In question 15, on the treatment of patients' eyes, the doctors were asked if, in addition to prescribing treatment and drugs, they would prescribe details of the methods to be used. Somewhat surprisingly, 41.3 per cent said they would always prescribe details of the method; 47.5 per cent said they would never prescribe the method. No explanation of these figures can be offered on the basis of medical as opposed to surgical specialisation as this activity was seen to be carried out 143 times, in both medical and surgical wards.

The staff nurses' score in this question was 60.7 per cent.

FIGURE 2 (SEE TABLE 8a)

STAFF NURSES' SCORES IN SCIENCE TEST AND DOCTORS'
EXPECTATIONS OF STAFF NURSES' KNOWLEDGE (GROUP C QUESTIONS)

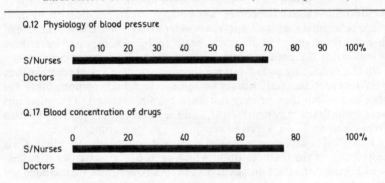

Q.12 Physiology of blood pressure

Q.17 Blood concentration of drugs

FIGURE 3 (TABLE 8b)

STAFF NURSES' SCORE IN SCIENCE TEST AND DOCTORS'
METHOD OF PRESCRIBING INTRAVENOUS FLUIDS

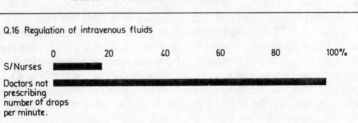

Q.16 Regulation of intravenous fluids

Doctors not
prescribing
number of drops
per minute.

FIGURE 4 (SEE TABLE 8c)

STAFF NURSES' SCORES IN SCIENCE TEST AND DOCTORS' EXPECTATIONS :
OF STAFF NURSES' ACTION IN INITIATING THE ACTIVITY
(GROUP C QUESTIONS)

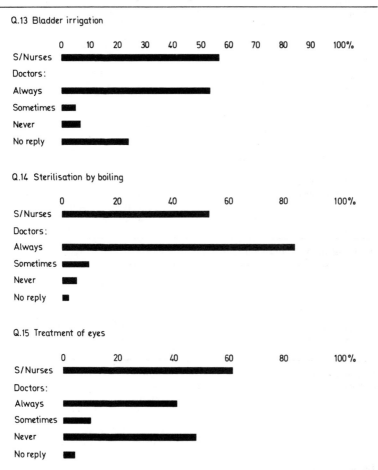

TABLE 8(a)

STAFF NURSES' SCORES IN SCIENCE TEST AND DOCTORS' EXPECTATIONS OF
STAFF NURSES' KNOWLEDGE (GROUP C QUESTIONS)

Question number, activity	Staff nurses' scores (N = 115) %	Doctors' expectations (N = 179) %
12. *Physiology of blood pressure*	70.14	58.93
17. *Blood concentration of drugs*	76.17	60.33

TABLE 8(b)

STAFF NURSES' SCORE IN SCIENCE TEST AND DOCTORS' METHOD OF
PRESCRIBING INTRAVENOUS FLUIDS

Question number, activity	Staff nurses' score (N = 115) %	Doctors prescribing drops per minute (N= 179) %
16. *Regulations of intravenous fluids*	16.52	1.67

TABLE 8(c)

STAFF NURSES' SCORES IN SCIENCE TEST AND DOCTORS' EXPECTATIONS OF STAFF
NURSES' ACTION IN ASSOCIATION WITH SPECIFIC ACTIVITIES OR SITUATIONS
(GROUP C QUESTIONS)

Question number, activity	Staff nurses (N = 115)	Doctors' expectations of whether staff nurses would initiate and take responsibility for activity (N = 179)			
	Scores %	Always %	Sometimes %	Never %	No reply %
13. *Bladder irrigation*	56.5	65.9	4.5	5.6	24.0
14. *Sterilisation by boiling*	52.9	84.4	9.5	4.5	1.7
15. *Treatment of eyes*	60.7	41.3	9.5	47.5	1.7
18. *Haemorrhage and pulse rate*	55.7	55.3	20.7	20.7	3.4
19. *Conversion imperial/metric measure*	58.8	70.4	7.3	18.4	3.9

3.2.2 Comparison of staff nurses' scores in the Science Test with the doctors' expectations of staff nurses knowledge, on items classified according to the sciences (Tables 9 to 13, pp. 61-64).

The items of activity in the questions in Groups A and B were classified according to the science from which they are derived. The nurses' scores and the doctors' expectations were compared by analysis of variance. The figures used for these calculations are shown in Tables 9 to 13. It was found that there was no significant difference between the staff nurses' scores and the doctors' expectations of the staff nurses' knowledge in any of the sciences.

This analysis was of interest as a possible guide to whether more emphasis should be pleased on any particular science subjects during the nursing education programme.

TABLE 9

STAFF NURSES' SCORES AND DOCTORS' EXPECTATIONS OF STAFF NURSES' KNOWLEDGE IN PHYSIOLOGY ITEMS (GROUP A and B QUESTIONS)

Question number	Item number	Activity	Staff nurses (N = 115) %	Doctors (N = 179) %
1	1	Getting a patient up	76.5	93.8
2	5	Surgical dressing technique	27.0	79.3
3	1	Urine testing	54.8	60.3
5	1	Oral hygiene	44.3	89.4
7	1	Abdominal paracentesis	72.2	93.8
8	3	Collection of specimens: microbiological	73.9	89.9
9	1	Pressure areas	29.6	97.8
9	3	Pressure areas	42.6	42.5
9	4	Pressure areas	89.6	36.9
9	5	Pressure areas	42.6	78.8

TABLE 10

STAFF NURSES' SCORES AND DOCTORS' EXPECTATIONS OF STAFF NURSES'
KNOWLEDGE IN MICROBIOLOGY ITEMS (GROUP A and B QUESTIONS)

Question number	Item number	Activity	Staff nurses (N = 115) %	Doctors (N = 179) %
2	1	Surgical dressing technique	24.3	84.9
2	2	Surgical dressing technique	80.0	88.8
2	3	Surgical dressing technique	36.5	57.0
2	4	Surgical dressing technique	80.9	82.7
2	6	Surgical dressing technique	80.9	87.2
3	5	Urine testing	91.3	72.6
4	3	Preparation for operation	89.6	68.2
6	1	Bathing patients: disinfection of bath	59.1	66.5
6	2	Bathing patients: disinfection of bath	89.6	85.5
6	3	Bathing patients: disinfection of bath	65.2	66.5
6	5	Bathing patients: disinfection of bath	44.3	72.1
7	3	Abdominal paracentesis	75.7	81.6
7	5	Abdominal paracentesis	38.3	83.8
8	1	Collection of specimens: microbiological	48.7	98.9
8	2	Collection of specimens: microbiological	53.9	82.1
8	4	Collection of specimens: microbiological	29.6	60.9
8	5	Collection of specimens: microbiological	71.3	91.6
8	6	Collection of specimens: microbiological	66.1	73.7
9	2	Pressure areas	69.6	99.4
10	2	Sterilisation by autoclaving	48.7	93.3
10	3	Sterilisation by autoclaving	59.1	92.7
10	4	Sterilisation by autoclaving	11.3	90.5
10	5	Sterilisation by autoclaving	66.1	91.6

TABLE 11

STAFF NURSES' SCORES AND DOCTORS' EXPECTATIONS OF STAFF NURSES' KNOWLEDGE
IN PATHOLOGY ITEMS (GROUP A and B QUESTIONS)

Question number	Item number	Activity	Staff nurses (N = 115) %	Doctors (N = 179) %
1	3	Getting a patient up	76.5	94.3
1	4	Getting a patient up	81.7	84.9
3	2	Urine testing	15.7	73.2
3	4	Urine testing	27.0	60.9
4	1	Preparation for operation	94.8	92.7
4	2	Preparation for operation	98.3	70.4
4	6	Preparation for operation	98.3	71.5
5	2	Oral hygiene	26.1	83.2
5	3	Oral hygiene	52.2	81.0
5	4	Oral hygiene	17.4	74.9
5	5	Oral hygiene	80.0	80.4
7	2	Abdominal paracentesis	46.1	79.3
7	4	Abdominal paracentesis	93.0	75.4
11	2	Weighing patients	60.9	45.8
11	6	Weighing patients	77.4	69.3

TABLE 12

STAFF NURSES' SCORES AND DOCTORS' EXPECTATIONS OF STAFF NURSES' KNOWLEDGE IN
PHARMACOLOGY ITEMS (GROUP A and B QUESTIONS)

Question number	Item number	Activity	Staff nurses (N = 115) %	Doctors (N = 179) %
1	2	Getting a patient up	60.9	83.8
4	4	Preparation for operation	93.9	86.1
4	5	Preparation for operation	95.6	83.8
6	4	Bathing patients: disinfection of bath	19.1	61.5
11	3	Weighing patients	87.8	49.7
11	4	Weighing patients	58.3	56.4
11	5	Weighing patients	85.2	71.5

TABLE 13

STAFF NURSES' SCORES AND DOCTORS' EXPECTATIONS OF STAFF NURSES' KNOWLEDGE
IN PHYSICS ITEMS (GROUP A and B QUESTIONS)

Question number	Item number	Activity	Staff nurses (N = 115) %	Doctors (N = 179) %
3	3	Urine testing	55.7	53.1
5	6	Oral hygiene	62.6	84.1
10	1	Sterilisation by autoclaving	32.2	91.6

3.3 COMPARISON OF DOCTORS' EXPECTATIONS OF THE STAFF NURSES' KNOWLEDGE, ACCORDING TO THE GRADE OF DOCTOR (Table 14, pp 67-68; Table 15, p. 69)

These analyses were based on the data obtained from the Doctors' Questionnaires only.

In the wards, staff nurses work with three grades of doctors: consultants, registrars and house officers. The more junior members of the medical staff spend more time in the wards than do the more senior staff. It seems, in fact, that the more senior they become the less time they actually spend in the wards.

It was decided to analyse the data to find out if there was any difference between the expectation of the more junior, less experienced doctors and their more senior colleagues, of whom most have postgraduate qualifications, and all have had considerably more experience of medical practice.

3.3.1 Comparison of doctors' expectations of the staff nurses' knowledge, in each question, according to the grade of doctor (Table 14, pp. 67-68; Table 15, p. 69)

The responses of the three groups of doctors to 13 questions were expressed as mean expectations and compared by analysis of variance. In the five questions in which an 'always/sometimes/never' answer was required, the responses were compared using the chi-square test.

The consultants' expectations of the staff nurses' knowledge were greater than those of the house officers in questions 1, 5 and 8, the difference in each case being significant. The subjects of these questions were: *question 1*, getting a patient up; question 5, oral hygiene; *question 8*, collection of specimens for microbiology.

The consultants' expectations of the staff nurses' knowledge were significantly greater than those of the registrars in question 19. In this question the doctors were asked if they expected staff nurses to take responsibility for the conversion of drug dosages from imperial to metric measures, or vice versa, if this was necessary.

The registrars' expectations of the staff nurses' knowledge were greater than those of the consultants in questions 4 and 9, the difference in each case being significant. These were on the subjects of: *question 4*, preparation of a patient for operation; *question 9*, the care of pressure areas.

The house officers' expectations of the staff nurses' knowledge were greater than those of the consultants in question 2 and 4. In *question 2*, on the subject of surgical dressing technique, the difference between the two groups was significant. In *question 4*, on the preparation of a patient for operation, it was highly significant.

The house officers' expectations of the staff nurses' knowledge were greater than those of the registrars in *question 7*, on the subject of abdominal paracentesis.

In the remainder of the comparisons there were no significant differences between the expectations of the three grades of doctors.

The differences between the three grades of doctor do not appear to conform to any pattern. From the findings of this study, it would seem that seniority is not a factor which has a significant influence on doctors' expectations of staff nurses' knowledge of the biological sciences or of the activities for which staff nurses are expected to take responsibility.

FIGURE 5 (SEE TABLE 14)

DOCTORS' EXPECTATIONS OF STAFF NURSES' KNOWLEDGE,
BY GRADE OF DOCTOR

Comparison of the mean number of items which the doctors expected the nurses to answer correctly in questions where the difference between the grades was significant.

Q.1 Getting a patient up (4 items)

Q.2 Surgical dressing technique (6 items)

Q.4 Preparation for operation (6 items)

Q.5 Oral hygiene (6 items)

Figure 5 Continued (Table 14)

Doctors' Expectations Of Staff Nurses' Knowledge,
By Grade Of Doctor

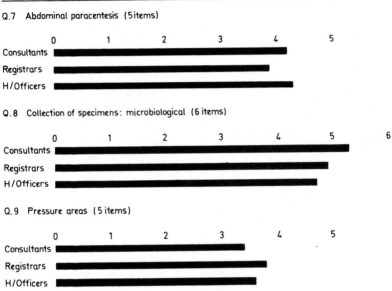

Q.7 Abdominal paracentesis (5 items)

Q.8 Collection of specimens: microbiological (6 items)

Q.9 Pressure areas (5 items)

Table 14

Doctors' Expectations Of Staff Nurses' Knowledge, By Grade Of Doctor:
Consultant (N = 72), Registrar (N = 45), House Officer (N = 62)

Question number, activity, respondents	Doctors' expectations Number of items							Totals	Means	Significant differences between groups F - ratios
	0	1	2	3	4	5	6			
1. *Getting a patient up*										
Consultants	2	2	2	8	58	-	-	262	3.64	Con/H.O.
Registrars	1	2	0	5	37	-	-	165	3.67	20.97
House Officers	0	0	11	14	37	-	-	212	3.42	df = 133 P<.01
2. *Surgical dressing technique*										
Consultants	13	0	0	2	6	18	33	318	4.42	H.O./Con.
Registrars	2	0	0	5	6	10	22	221	4.90	6.56
House Officers	1	0	1	2	6	21	31	323	5.21	df = 133 P<.05

TABLE 14 CONTINUED

3. *Urine testing*
Consultants	10	6	5	12	10	29	-	237	3.29
Registrars	7	4	4	8	5	17	-	141	3.13
House Officers	8	6	5	13	10	20	-	195	3.15

4. *Preparation for operation*
Consultants	9	4	5	10	11	13	20	273	3.79	Reg./Con.
Registrars	0	0	5	5	6	12	17	211	4.69	6.59
House Officers	1	2	4	10	12	14	19	272	4.50	df = 116 $P<.05$;

H.O./Con.
6.96
df = 133 $P<.01$

5. *Oral Hygiene*
Consultants	1	1	2	4	4	13	47	380	5.28	Con/H.O.
Registrars	2	0	2	3	5	11	22	220	4.89	9.75
House Officers	0	3	7	6	7	16	23	281	4.53	df = 133 $P<.01$

6. *Bathing patients: disinfection of bath*
Consultants	3	5	11	6	11	36	-	269	3.74
Registrars	1	4	8	8	4	20	-	160	3.56
House Officers	5	6	9	12	9	21	-	201	3.24

7. *Abdominal paracentesis*
Consultants	1	3	3	9	15	41	-	301	4.18	H.O./Reg.
Registrars	1	3	2	10	8	21	-	174	3.87	4.17
House Officers	0	0	2	11	16	33	-	266	4.29	df = 106 $P<.05$

8. *Collection of specimens: microbiological*
Consultants	0	0	1	3	11	19	38	378	5.25	Con./H.O.
Registrars	0	0	1	4	8	19	13	219	4.87	8.4
House Officers	0	1	2	4	16	22	17	293	7.70	df = 133 $P<.01$

9. *Pressure areas*
Consultants	1	0	9	32	21	9	-	243	3.38	Reg./Con.
Registrars	0	0	5	13	13	14	-	171	3.80	4.29
House Officers	0	0	10	18	22	12	-	222	3.58	df = 116 $P<.05$

10. *Sterilisation by autoclaving*
Consultants	4	1	0	0	1	66	-	335	4.65
Registrars	3	0	0	0	2	40	-	208	4.62
House Officers	4	0	0	4	3	51	-	279	4.50

11. *Weighing patients*
Consultants	15	1	9	8	10	15	14	242	3.36	
Registrars	5	3	6	10	5	2	14	159	3.53	
House Officers	9	5	7	6	12	6	17	217	3.50	

12. *Physiology of blood pressure*
Consultants	5	13	14	19	21	-	-	182	2.53
Registrars	5	10	8	10	12	-	-	104	2.31
House Officers	10	8	17	14	13	-	-	136	2.19

17. *Blood concentration of drugs*
Consultants	8	7	20	23	14	-	-	172	2.39
Registrars	7	6	11	11	10	-	-	101	2.24
House Officers	4	6	19	17	16	-	-	159	2.56

TABLE 15

DOCTORS' EXPECTATIONS OF STAFF NURSES' ACTIONS IN ASSOCIATION WITH
SPECIFIC ACTIVITIES AND SITUATIONS, BY GRADE OF DOCTOR: CONSULTANT (N = 72),
REGISTRAR (N = 45), HOUSE OFFICER (N = 62)

Question number, activity, respondents	Doctors' expectations of whether staff nurses would initiate and take responsibility for activity				Significant differences between groups x^2
	Always %	Sometimes %	Never %	No Answer %	
13. *Bladder irrigation*					
Consultants	54.17	2.78	2.78	40.28	
Registrars	66.67	6.67	8.89	17.78	
House Officers	79.03	4.84	6.45	9.68	
14. *Sterilisation by boiling*					
Consultants	86.11	8.33	4.17	1.39	
Registrars	82.22	11.11	4.44	2.22	
House Officers	83.87	9.68	4.84	1.61	
15. *Treatment of eyes*					
Consultants	38.89	12.50	47.22	1.39	
Registrars	40.0	8.89	51.11		
House Officers	45.16	6.45	45.16	3.22	
18. *Haemorrhage and pulse rate*					
Consultants	51.39	23.61	19.44	5.56	
Registrars	64.44	15.56	17.78	2.22	
House Officers	53.23	20.97	24.19	1.61	
19. *Conversion of drug dosages*					
Consultants	76.39	5.56	13.90	4.17	Con./Reg.
Registrars	51.11	8.89	33.33	6.67	$x^2 = 9.43$
House Officers	77.42	8.06	12.90	1.61	$P < .05$

3.3.2 Comparison of doctors' expectations of the staff nurses' knowledge, according to the form in which the questions were presented in the Doctors' Questionnaire (Table 16).

Three types of question (Groups A, B and C) were used in the Doctors' Questionnaire, each of which provided them with a different amount of detailed information. It was decided to compare the mean number of responses of all the doctors to the three types of question.

The responses which were used in relation to the Group C questions, which asked for an 'always/sometimes/never' answer, were those which indicated that the doctors expected staff nurses to initiate or take responsibility for an activity.

When the differences between the mean number of responses to each type of question were tested for significance by analysis of variance, the only one found to be significant was the difference between Group A and Group C questions (F = 5.55, df 14). The doctors had greater expectations in relation to the more detailed questions in Group A than in relation to the more general questions in Group C.

TABLE 16

THE DOCTORS' AFFIRMATIVE RESPONSES TO THE
THREE DIFFERENT TYPES OF QUESTION

Type of question	Sum of doctors' responses	Mean number of responses
Group A Questions 1-7	981	140.14
Group B Questions 8-11	543	135.75
Group C Questions 12-19	796	99.5

3.4 DISCUSSION OF THE FINDINGS

The findings of the study indicate that doctors expect staff nurses to have more knowledge of the biological sciences than was demonstrated by the staff nurses. From the review of the literature, it would seem that nurses should assume that they will be asked to take over more and more activities which were previously carried out by doctors.

Although the present study was not concerned with the staff nurses' technical abilities, the findings raise doubts as to whether there is a similar gap between the staff nurses' performance and the doctors' expectations of their performance. If it is believed that the staff nurse's knowledge is related to her technical ability it is necessary to consider what action should be taken to bring this knowledge and the doctors' expectations of this knowledge into closer proximity.

There are two ways in which this could be done.

1. The doctors could adopt a more realistic view of the staff nurses' abilities.

2. The staff nurses could be educated to a level which is consistent with the doctors' expectations.

To take no action would be to perpetuate the potentially hazardous situation for the patients which these findings reveal.

The development of a more realistic view on the part of the doctors would necessitate a radical rethinking, on their part, of the role and functions of nurses. From the literature it would seem that doctors are rethinking their own function, but this is generally along the lines of trying to relieve themselves of activities and responsibilities which they would like taken over by others.

This seems to be an unlikely development.

A more likely method of bridging the gap between the staff nurses' knowledge and the doctors' expectations would be to raise the educational level of nurses with respect to the biological sciences.

In the medical journals, doctors referred frequently to the fact that nurses need to acquire technical skills. In the Doctors' Questionnaire, this somewhat narrow view of nursing was extended to include the taking of responsibility and the initiating of activities by nurses. These two aspects of the abilities which staff nurses are expected to possess seem to be essential components of knowledge to be acquired during a professional education. They depend on the acquisition of 'facts', together with the ability to assess the relative importance of 'facts' and to use them in particular situations.

In an article entitled 'Teaching and learning', Oakeshott (1967) describes the development of 'knowing' as part of the educational process:

> Now, these abilities of various kinds and dimensions which constitute what we may be said to know will be found to be conjunctions of what is called 'information' and what I shall call 'judgement'.

Of information he goes on to say that 'it is the explicit ingredient of knowledge' and that it consists of facts which can be itemised. These are necessary as a basis for 'rule-like propositions' which enable appropriate action to be taken:

> They may be items of information which must be known as a condition of being able to perform; or they may constitute the criterion by means of which a performance may be known to be incorrect...

This is the area of ability upon which staff nurses were tested and the doctors asked to express their expectations of the staff nurses' knowledge in the group A and B questions.

The group C questions in the Doctors' Questionnaire were more in the area of what Oakeshott describes as 'judgement'. He says:

Before any concrete skill or ability can appear, information is partnered by 'judgement', 'know *how*' must be added to the 'know *what*' of information.

...Information has to be used, and it does not itself indicate how, on any occasion, it should be used. What is required in addition to information is knowledge which enables us to interpret it, to decide upon its relevance, to recognise what rule to apply and to discover what action permitted by the rule should, in the circumstances, be performed, knowledge (in short) capable of carrying us acorss the wide open spaces, to be found in every ability, where no rule runs. For rules are always disjunctive. They specify only an act or a conclusion of a certain general kind and they never relieve us of the necessity of choice...

'Judgement', then, is not to be recognised as merely information of another sort; its deliverances cannot be itemized... and they are neither remembered nor forgotten. It is, for example, all that is contained in what has been called 'the unspecifiable art of scientific enquiry' without which 'the articulate contents of scientific knowledge' remains unintelligible.

Fact, or information which is the word used in this context, can be taught and the student can have something specific which can be learned from the teacher and from textbooks. This is an area of knowledge which can be tested by examination. Judgement, on the other hand, Oakeshott maintains, cannot be explicitly taught. It is something which the students learn from the attitudes of their teachers and from the examples they are given by practitioners in the situation.

It is clear from his argument that Oakeshott considers that this less tangible ingredient of knowledge, judgement, is essential for people to make the best use of the information at their disposal. Judgement is needed by doctors in making a diagnosis; by nurses in deciding to initiate an activity; by teachers in selecting, organising and presenting information.

There is a considerable overlap in the functions of nurses and doctors and, as Scott (1965) indicated, it is important that a dynamic state in relation to 'who does what' should be maintained. If there is an overlap in functions there must also be an area of information which is common to the two professions.

The uses to which the two professions put their common body of information is of some interest in relation both to the provision of effective medical and nursing services and in the planning of medical and nursing education.

It was said previously that nurses spend considerably more time in contact with the patients in the wards than doctors do. It was suggested by one writer that a generous estimate of the amount of time which a doctor spends in contact with a patient in a week would be of the order of one hour.

Although each individual nurse works on the basis of an eight hour day, a continuity of nursing service is provided by the nursing team. This means that the series of registered nurses in charge of the patients receive a continuous stream of information about the patients which is the result of observations made by the individual members of the nursing team.

Figure 6 illustrates some of the decisions, or judgements, made by nurses and doctors using information which is acquired originally from the general practitioner, the patient and the patient's family.

FIGURE 6

USE OF INFORMATION BY NURSES AND DOCTORS

HOSPITAL

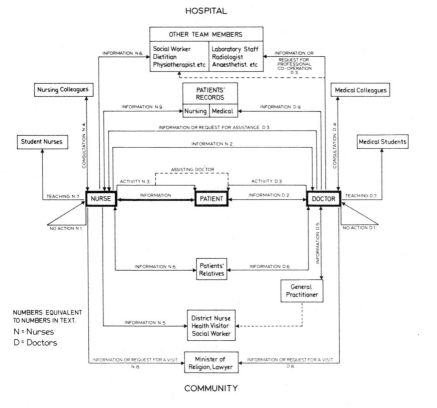

COMMUNITY

In describing the diagram 'the nurse' applies to a registered nurse working the position of staff nurse or ward sister and is in charge of a ward.

The nurse decides what to do with the information she receives in the light of her knowledge of the patient's provisional or final diagnosis and the aims of the investigations and medical treatments prescribed by the doctor. The nurse may decide that the information:

1. is not of immediate relevance and should be recorded for possible future reference, or that it is confidential and cannot be given to others without the patient's permission;

2. will be of value to the doctor and will assist him in making medical decisions;

3. necessitates the initiation of nursing activity without consultation with the doctor;

4. will be of value when consulting with a nursing colleague and/or could assist other members of the patient care team, for example, dietitians, social workers, physiotherapists, in making decisions within their sphere of patient care;

5. will be of value to the health visitor, the district nurse, the social worker, when the patient is discharged;

6. will be of value to the patient's relatives, for example, in their planning for the patient's discharge from hospital or for his prolonged stay;

7. will be of value to her in teaching student and pupil nurses and in supervising the work of the nursing team:

8. may be of value in any discussion with the patient's minister of religion or legal adviser;

9. should be recorded in the patient's notes.

The nurse may also be involved in further action, resulting from her decision to pass on information.

She is frequently responsible for ensuring that the treatment prescribed by the doctor is given, that a diagnostic test is carried out, and that information is communicated to the patient and to his relatives, for example, that he is ready to go home.

If the doctor prescribes and carries out the treatment or test himself, the nurse is usually involved in ensuring that the patient and the equipment are prepared and that a nurse accompanies the doctor to assist him and the patient during the treatment.

The doctor's original decision, in the hospital situation, is to admit the patient. This is based on information which he has received from the general practitioner and from his examination of the patient as an out-patient; or on the basis of his examination of the patient who arrives at the hospital as an emergency.

When the patient has been admitted to the hospital, the doctor's sources of information are his direct contact with the patient, the results of diagnostic tests, and the nurse.

The doctor, like the nurse, has a number of choices regarding what he will do with the information which he receives from the nurse. He may decide that the information:

1. is not of immediate relevance and should be recorded for future reference, or that it is confidential and cannot be given to others without the patient's permission

2. necessitates communication with the patient: to examine, to give treatment, to convey information, for example, regarding treatment or discharge;

3. will be used in making a diagnosis or in prescribing; he may

prescribe treatment, diagnostic tests, or that the patient can be discharged from hospital;

4. will be of value while consulting with a medical colleague or other member of the patient care team;

5. should be communicated to the patient's general practitioner;

6. will be of value to the patient's relatives in planning for the patient's discharge from hospital or for his prolonged stay;

7. will be of value in teaching medical students;

8. may be of value in any discussion with the patient's minister of religion or legal adviser;

9. should be recorded in the patient's case notes.

From this description it can be seen that the work of the nurse in charge of the ward is largely that of a decision-maker and communicator; if this series of activities is multiplied by the number of patients in the ward, it is very doubtful whether she will have time personally to participate in the giving of patient care.

The crucial stage in the series of decisions made by the nurse is the point at which she decides whether information is of significance and, if so, to whom. This is how she *enables* others to contribute to the care of the patients, and from which a number of cycles of events begins.

It was not intended, in this study, to attempt to define the level of knowledge of the biological sciences required by nurses. However, some indication of this can be deduced from the different ways in which doctors and nurses use their knowledge of these sciences. It would seem that nurses use their knowledge in two ways. One is in giving direct patient care and the other in recognising and passing on to others, information which will contribute to their decision-making.

The doctor adds the information which he received from the nurse to that which he has acquired from other sources, for example, from laboratory reports, X-rays, and of course, the patient. He collates this more detailed information in order to make a differential diagnosis and to prescribe treatment.

It would seem that generally the nurse requires to have knowledge of the same sciences as the doctor, over the same range of material derived from these sciences, but not to the same depth, as she is not responsible for making the final diagnosis or prescribing the medical treatment.

4. Findings: Staff Nurses and Student Nurses

4.1 INTRODUCTION

This section is concerned with the knowledge of the biological sciences shown by staff nurses, and by student nurses at different stages of their training and experience, as demonstrated by their scores in the Science Test. The results have also been related to the observations of nurses' activities in the wards, which were carried out during the initial stages of the study.

Three schools of nursing were involved and the programming of the theory taught in the classroom was different in each. No attempt has been made to relate the Science Test scores of the students with the theory as it was taught in the curriculum of their own schools. The stage at which the students were given the theoretical content of their course was irrelevant in the present study because the Science Test questions were based solely on activities which the students were seen to perform in the wards.

It has been suggested in Chapter 1 that the mass of theory which student nurses are expected and assumed to absorb is ill-defined, that the manner in which they acquire and learn to apply such knowledge in the clinical situation is unstructured and appears to be haphazard. The knowledge which they require in order to perform safely the activities which they actually carry out at different stages of their training has not been investigated, and a satisfactory method of assessing their knowledge at different stages of their training, in association with the activities which they perform, has not been devised.

This study is concerned with one area of the students' knowledge (the biological sciences) in relation to the activities which they were seen to perform at different stages of their training. Whether they should have been performing these activities was fortunately not the concern of this study.

In this section, comparison will be made between the Science Test scores obtained by staff nurses, third year, second year, and first year students: their total scores on the whole Science Test; their scores in each of the questions which were related to specific nursing activities; and their scores on items within each question, classified according to the sciences.

The relationship will be shown between the score of each group of nurses in the Science Test and the frequency with which they were seen to carry out the nursing activities on which the test questions were based.

4.2 COMPARISON OF THE SCORES OF EACH GROUP OF NURSES IN THE SCIENCE TEST

4.2.1 Comparison of total scores in the Science Test: the mean score of each group of nurses compared with the mean score of each of the other groups (Table 17, p. 78).

Comparison was made of the results from 18 questions out of the 19 which comprised the whole test. Question 7 was omitted because it was presented to staff nurses and 3rd year students only, these being the only nurses who were observed to carry out the activities on which the question was based.

The total score obtainable in the 18 questions was 95. Table 17 shows the mean score and the standard deviation from the mean for each group of nurses.

Analysis of variance was used to test the significance of differences between the mean scores of the four groups (Garrett, 1958 a). All the differences were found to be highly significant, and in each case the more senior group had the higher mean score. Differences between the standard deviations were not significant.

These results were to some extent predictable: the staff nurses, at the upper end of the scale, had completed their course of study and were in at least their fourth year of nursing practice, and there was approximately one year's difference between the length of time each of the student nurse groups had been in training.

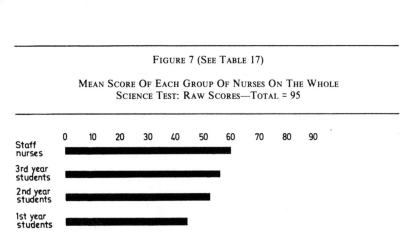

FIGURE 7 (SEE TABLE 17)

MEAN SCORE OF EACH GROUP OF NURSES ON THE WHOLE SCIENCE TEST: RAW SCORES—TOTAL = 95

TABLE 17

ANALYSIS OF TOTAL SCORES IN SCIENCE TEST, FOR EACH GROUP OF NURSES:
STANDARD DEVIATION, MEAN SCORE AND SIGNIFICANCE OF DIFFERENCE
BETWEEN MEAN SCORES

Group	Standard deviation	Mean score (Total = 95)	Significant difference between means		
			Groups	F - ratio	Significance level
Staff nurses (N = 115)	10.14	60.03	S.N./3rd year	7.9	P < .01
			S.N./2nd year	266.6	P < .01
			S.N./1st year	138.8	P < .01
3rd year students (N = 136)	10.06	56.43	3rd year/2nd year	15.8	P < .01
			3rd year/1st year	92.9	P < .01
2nd year students (N = 143)	9.35	51.80	2nd year/1st year	40.1	P < .01
1st year students (N = 138)	11.28	43.94			

4.2.2 Comparison of nurses' scores in each question in the Science Test: the mean score of each group of nurses compared with the mean score of each of the other groups (Table 18 pp. 87/88; Table 19, p. 90).

Considerable differences were found between the mean scores of the groups, in individual questions. These differences were tested for significance by analysis of variance.

Tables 18 and 19 show the result of these analyses. In each question six comparisons were made between the mean scores of the four groups.

4.2.2.1 *Comparison of the nurses' mean score in each question in the Science Test, according to their years of experience* (Table 18, pp. 87/88/89; Table 19, p. 90).

One year's difference between the groups:
Staff nurses and third year students (19 questions). The difference between their mean scores was highly significant in three questions and significant in one, the staff nurses in each case showing more knowledge than the third year students. In the remaining 15 questions the differences between the mean scores were not significant.

Third year and second year students (18 questions). The difference between the mean scores was highly significant in two questions and significant in one. In two of these the third year students had the higher mean score and in one the second year students' score was higher. In the remaining 15 questions the differences between the mean scores were not significant.

Second year and first year students (18 questions). There was a considerably greater number of differences between the mean scores of second and first year students than between the other groups. In eight questions the difference was highly significant and in two questions significant. In each of these questions, the mean score of the second year students was higher than that of the first year students. In the remaining eight questions the differences between the mean scores were not significant.

Two years' difference between the groups:
Staff nurses and second year students (18 questions). The difference between the mean scores was highly significant in eight questions and significant in one. In seven questions the mean score of the staff nurses was higher and in one question the second year students scored higher. In the remaining nine questions the differences between the mean scores were not significant.

Third and first year students (18 questions). The difference between the mean scores of the two groups was highly significant in eleven questions and significant in two questions. In each of these questions the mean score of the third year students was higher than that of the first year students. In the remaining five questions the differences between the mean scores were not significant.

Three years' difference between the groups:

Staff nurses and first year students (18 questions). The difference between the mean scores of the two groups was highly significant in 12 questions and significant in one question. In each case the staff nurses' mean score was the higher. In the remaining five questions the differences between the mean scores were not significant.

4.2.2.2 *Comparison of the nurses' mean score in each question in the Science Test, according to the number of significant differences between the groups* (Table 18, pp. 87-89; Table 19, p. 90; Table 28, p. 99).

In questions 4, 11, and 19, five of the six tests carried out on the differences between mean scores were found to be highly significant and in each of these the more senior group had a higher mean score.

Question 4: preparing patients for operation under general anaesthetic: The difference between the mean scores of staff nurses and third year students was the only one which was not significant. From Table 18 it will be seen that there were six items in the question and that the mean scores of the groups increased gradually with each year of seniority, from 4.39 for first year students to 5.70 for staff nurses.

A similar pattern emerged in relation to the frequency with which this activity was observed in the wards. Of the total number of times this activity was seen to be carried out, 38.1 per cent was by staff nurses and 19.1 per cent by first year students, that is, the group with most background knowledge of the activity carried it out most frequently (Table 28).

Question 11: reasons for weighing patients in hospital. The difference between the mean scores of third and second year students was the only one which was not significant.

There were six items in this question and the mean scores of the groups increased with each year of seniority from 3.04 for first year students to 4.30 for staff nurses (Table 18). The pattern of the frequency of observations of this activity in the wards was somewhat different from that of the scores. Table 28 shows that, of the total number of times this activity was seen to be carried out, 72.2 per cent was by staff nurses; 2.9 per cent by third year students; 8.9 per cent by second year students, and 15.9 per cent by first year students.

It would seem from this that, when the staff nurses do not carry out the activity themselves, it is not considered essential for the nurses to whom the activity is assigned to have background knowledge about the task, otherwise the staff nurses, who appear to have such knowledge, would presumably pass it on to them.

Question 19: conversion from imperial to metric measure of some commonly prescribed doses of drugs. The difference between the mean scores of the staff nurses and third year students was the only one which was not significant.

The mean scores of the student groups showed a sharp decline from

3.12 in the third year to 1.38 in the first year. The total score obtainable in this question was 6 (Table 18).

During the period of observation in the wards it was noted that the administration of drugs sometimes required nurses to convert doses from imperial to metric measure. The observer was alerted to this as a nursing activity when asked by a student to check the dose of a drug which she had converted. It was not possible to find out how often this was done and by whom, but it was noted that the drugs and doses included in the question were sometimes prescribed by the doctors in imperial and sometimes in metric measure. It was also noted that the pharmacy in each hospital used only one scale of measurement for each drug supplied to the wards.

The pattern of frequency with which activities associated with this question were observed in the wards was the same as that of the scores (Table 28). Although the mean scores seemed to be remarkably low, the nurses with most knowledge carried out the activities most frequently.

In questions 6, 9 and 14, none of the six tests carried out on the differences between mean scores was found to be significant.

Question 6: bathing patients and disinfection of the bath. This question was included to represent a variety of situations in the wards in which the use of chemical disinfectants was the only means of treating equipment contaminated by infected discharges from patients. If the use of disinfectants was not effective, there was a risk to the patients of cross-infection.

First year students were seen to carry out this activity most frequently (Table 28). It would seem from this that the students had learned the microbiological and pharmacological principles associated with this activity at an early stage in their training programme and had retained this knowledge.

Question 9: the care of pressure areas to prevent the development of decubitus ulcers. This question was included because of the high frequency with which the activity was observed in the wards (4319 times). Staff nurses carried it out 378 times (8.8 per cent of the total); third years students 790 times (18.3 per cent); second year students 971 times (22.5 per cent); and first year students 2180 times (50.5 per cent). Although this is an essential part of the nursing care of patients who are confined to bed the observer had the impression that, at least as far as first year students were concerned, it was a largely routine, non-selective activity. There were stated times of the day when 'the back round' was done. It was not uncommon to hear the junior night nurse (first year student) ask patients to go to bed to have their 'back rubbed'. If junior students are introduced to the care of pressure areas in this somewhat meaningless routine way they may fail to see the importance of the background theory upon which the activity depends.

The fact that the students learned to think of this procedure simply as rubbing an area of skin may have dulled their sensitivity to the wider issues involved in caring for the skin of selected patients, for whom the treatment could be of considerable importance.

There were five items in the question and the mean score was 2.70 for all groups except third year students for whom it was 2.90. (Table 18).

Question 14: sterilisation by boiling. At the time when these data were collected, boiling water sterilisers were used for a considerable variety of equipment in all the wards in which observations of activities were carried out. In the intervening period other methods of sterilisation have been introduced for at least some of the equipment used in the wards.

There were six items in the question and the mean scores increased gradually from 2.90 for first year students to 3.10 for staff nurses (Table 18). The observations of this activity did not form the same pattern: second and third year students carried out the activity more frequently than did staff nurses and first year students. It would seem therefore that the ward sisters or staff nurses who assign nursing activities to the different nursing personnel do not always consider it necessary for the group carrying out the activity most frequently to be the one with the most knowledge of the associated physics and microbiology.

The remaining 12 questions showed a varied number of significant differences between the mean scores of the four groups of nurses.

Table 19 shows that of the 18 questions presented to the four groups of nurses there were four significant differences in five questions, three significant differences in three questions, two significant differences in three questions, and only one in one question. In question 7, which was presented to staff nurses and third year students only, the staff nurses' mean score was higher than that of the third year students. The difference was highly significant.

With the exception of questions 6, 9 and 14, which have already been discussed, and two other questions, 10 and 12, there was some consistency in where the significant differences between mean scores occurred in the remaining 13 questions. Significant differences were found between mean scores of first year students and those of staff nurses and third year students. In each case the mean score of first year students was lower than the mean scores of the other two groups. In eight of these 13 questions, second year students had a significantly higher mean score than first year students, and in eight questions the mean score of staff nurses was significantly higher than that of second year students. In the remaining comparisons, that is, between staff nurses and third year students and between third and second year students, there were few significant differences and these showed no consistent pattern.

The same consistency is not apparent in relation to the frequency with which each group was seen to carry out activities associated with the questions asked. In five of the 13 questions in which first year students had the lowest mean score, these students carried out the highest percentage of associated activities, that is, questions 1, 3, 5, 8 and 18 (Table 28).

FIGURE 8 (SEE TABLE 18)

MEAN SCORE OF EACH GROUP OF NURSES IN EACH QUESTION IN THE SCIENCE TEST

Comparison of the mean number of items answered correctly by each group of nurses in questions where the difference was significant

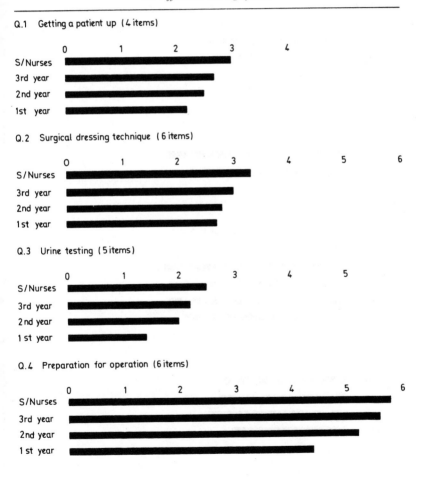

FIGURE 8 CONTINUED (SEE TABLE 18)

MEAN SCORE OF EACH GROUP OF NURSES IN EACH QUESTION IN THE
SCIENCE TEST

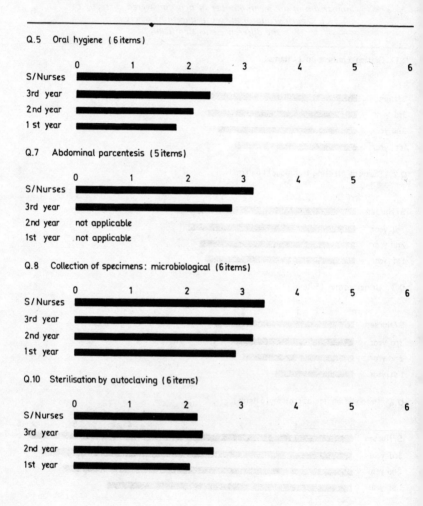

FIGURE 8 CONTINUED (SEE TABLE 18)

MEAN SCORE OF EACH GROUP OF NURSES IN EACH QUESTION IN THE
SCIENCE TEST

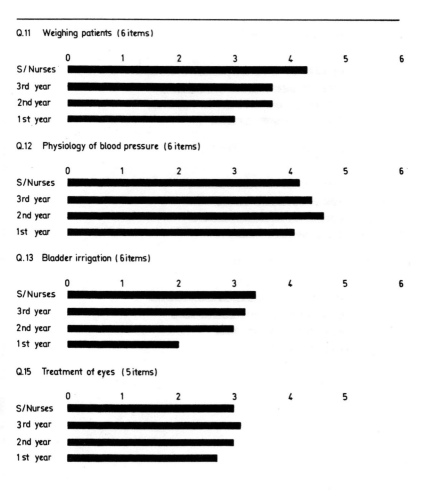

Q.11   Weighing patients (6 items)

Q.12   Physiology of blood pressure (6 items)

Q.13   Bladder irrigation (6 items)

Q.15   Treatment of eyes (5 items)

FIGURE 8 CONTINUED (SEE TABLE 18)

MEAN SCORE OF EACH GROUP OF NURSES IN EACH QUESTION IN THE
SCIENCE TEST

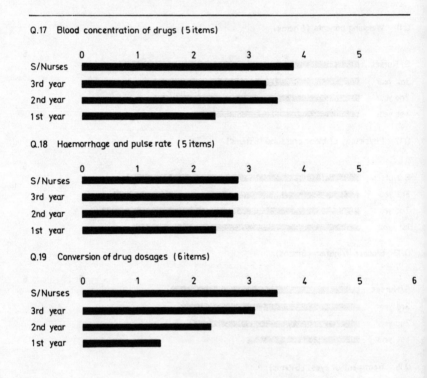

TABLE 18

SCORES OF EACH GROUP OF NURSES IN EACH QUESTION IN SCIENCE TEST:
MEAN SCORES AND SIGNIFICANT DIFFERENCES BETWEEN MEAN SCORES:
STAFF NURSES (N = 115), 3rd YEAR STUDENTS (N = 136), 2nd YEAR STUDENTS (N = 143),
1st YEAR STUDENTS (N = 138)

Question number, activity, respondents	Scores: Number of items correct							Totals	Means	Significant differences between means	
	0	1	2	3	4	5	6			Groups	Level
1. *Getting a patient up*										S.N./2	$P<.01$
Staff nurses	5	5	24	37	44	-	-	340	2.95	S.N./1	$P<.01$
3rd year students	6	10	39	44	37	-	-	368	2.71	3/1	$P<.01$
2nd year students	6	23	36	49	29	-	-	358	2.50	2/1	$P<.01$
1st year students	11	27	42	42	16	-	-	301	2.18		
2. *Surgical dressing technique*											
Staff nurses	2	9	16	40	27	16	5	379	3.30	S.N./2	$P<.01$
3rd year students	4	15	22	47	28	18	2	414	3.04	S.N./1	$P<.01$
2nd year students	5	17	32	51	23	14	1	402	2.81	3/1	$P<.05$
1st year students	4	24	31	37	31	10	1	377	2.73		
3. *Urine testing*											
Staff nurses	2	26	31	35	16	5	-	282	2.45	S.N./2	$P<.01$
3rd year students	3	30	51	32	18	2	-	310	2.21	S.N./1	$P<.01$
2nd year students	16	26	54	30	16	1	-	293	2.04	3/1	$P<.01$
1st year students	36	40	35	21	5	1	-	198	1.43	2/1	$P<.01$
4. *Preparation for operation*										S.N./2	$P<.01$
Staff nurses	0	1	2	2	1	13	96	656	5.70	S.N./1	$P<.01$
3rd year students	0	0	1	1	9	28	97	763	5.60	3/2	$P<.01$
2nd year students	4	2	1	9	18	24	85	739	5.17	3/1	$P<0.1$
1st year students	2	5	14	17	24	30	46	606	4.39	2/1	$P<.01$
5. *Oral hygiene*											
Staff nurses	8	10	31	28	25	9	4	325	2.83	S.N./3	$P<.05$
3rd year students	13	26	35	27	25	9	1	328	2.41	S.N./2	$P<.01$
2nd year students	17	38	35	27	22	2	2	299	2.09	S.N./1	$P<.01$
1st year students	27	36	36	21	11	7	0	250	1.80	3/1	$P<.01$
6. *Bathing patients: disinfection of bath*											
Staff nurses	1	6	21	32	35	20	-	384	3.34		
3rd year students	1	3	37	34	39	19	-	430	3.16		
2nd year students	0	5	25	38	57	18	-	487	3.41		
1st year students	2	6	18	42	50	20	-	468´	3.39		
7. *Abdominal paracentesis*											
Staff nurses	3	9	12	40	35	16	-	373	3.24	S.N./3	$P<.01$
3rd year students	7	6	33	52	30	8	-	388	2.85		
8. *Collection of specimens: (microbiological)*											
Staff nurses	2	8	24	23	27	24	7	395	3.43	S.N./1	$P<.01$
3rd year students	3	9	29	38	33	20	4	437	3.20	3/1	$P<.95$
2nd year students	2	17	27	38	33	22	4	451	3.15		
1st year students	9	15	30	36	31	13	4	396	2.86		

TABLE 18 CONTINUED

SCORES OF EACH GROUP OF NURSES IN EACH QUESTION IN SCIENCE TEST:
MEAN SCORES AND SIGNIFICANT DIFFERENCES BETWEEN MEAN SCORES:
STAFF NURSES (N = 115), 3rd YEAR STUDENTS (N = 136), 2nd YEAR STUDENTS (N = 143),
1st YEAR STUDENTS (N = 138)

Question number, activity, respondents	Scores: Number of items correct							Totals	Means	Significant differences between means	
	0	1	2	3	4	5	6			Groups	Level
9. Pressure areas											
Staff nurses	4	9	41	32	17	12	-	315	2.70		
3rd year students	4	5	37	56	26	8	-	391	2.90		
2nd year students	3	17	36	55	25	7	-	389	2.70		
1st year students	3	10	44	55	24	2	-	369	2.70		
10. Sterilisation by autoclaving											
Staff nurses	13	16	34	35	16	1	0	258	2.24	2/1	P<.05
3rd year students	26	17	28	33	26	4	2	308	2.26		
2nd year students	9	19	41	42	25	7	0	362	2.50		
1st year students	26	26	28	32	17	8	1	292	2.10		
11. Weighing patients										S.N./3	P<.01
Staff nurses	2	0	5	15	40	39	14	494	4.30	S.N./2	P<.01
3rd year students	8	1	5	34	49	36	3	507	3.73	S.N./1	P<.01
2nd year students	4	1	8	40	61	28	1	527	3.68	3/1	P<.01
1st year students	7	13	23	38	40	16	1	419	3.04	2/1	P<.01
12. Physiology of blood pressure											
Staff nurses	2	1	9	19	31	34	19	484	4.21	S.N./2	P<.01
3rd year students	3	0	7	14	45	47	20	591	4.35	3/2	P<.05
2nd year students	2	0	4	17	29	59	32	662	4.63	2/1	P<.01
1st year students	9	2	10	21	33	34	29	561	4.07		
13. Bladder irrigation											
Staff nurses	4	11	20	24	23	23	10	390	3.39	S.N./2	P<.05
3rd year students	2	15	32	27	30	20	10	440	3.23	S.N./1	P<.01
2nd year students	14	17	22	29	37	16	8	424	2.97	3/1	P<.01
1st year students	32	28	33	20	10	11	4	273	1.98	2/1	P<.01
14. Sterilisation by boiling											
Staff nurses	4	11	24	25	30	15	6	365	3.10		
3rd year students	5	11	31	40	37	11	1	402	3.00		
2nd year students	1	17	39	49	28	7	2	401	2.80		
1st year students	4	13	34	41	32	11	3	405	2.90		
15. Treatment of eyes											
Staff nurses	4	7	15	51	31	7	-	349	3.03	S.N./1	P<.05
3rd year students	1	7	24	62	35	7	-	416	3.05	3/1	P<.01
2nd year students	4	8	29	59	36	7	-	422	2.95	2/1	P<.05
1st year students	7	16	34	45	30	6	-	369	2.67		
17. Blood concentration of drugs											
Staff nurses	2	2	7	29	42	33	-	436	3.79	S.N./3	P<.01
3rd year students	10	4	16	35	51	20	-	445	3.27	S.N./1	P<.01
2nd year students	11	4	10	38	41	39	-	497	3.48	3/1	P<.01
1st year students	30	10	22	34	30	12	-	336	2.43	2/1	P<.01

TABLE 18 CONTINUED

Question number, activity, respondents	Scores Number of items correct							Totals	Means	Significant differences between means	
	0	1	2	3	4	5	6			Groups	Level
18. *Haemorrhage and pulse rate*											
Staff nurses	3	8	37	39	19	9	-	320	2.78	S.N./1	$P < .01$
3rd year students	5	11	32	50	31	7	-	384	2.82	3/1	$P < .01$
2nd year students	7	17	40	40	30	9	-	382	2.67		
1st year students	13	26	30	43	19	7	-	326	2.36		
19. *Conversion of drug dosages*										S.N./2	$P < .01$
Staff nurses	21	6	7	17	12	25	27	406	3.53	S.N./1	$P < .01$
3rd year students	28	14	16	15	13	19	31	424	3.12	3/2	$P < .01$
2nd year students	44	25	12	19	15	11	17	323	2.26	3/1	$P < .01$
1st year students	81	15	8	7	9	5	13	191	1.38	2/1	$P < .01$

16. *Regulation of intravenous fluids*	No answer	Wrong	Right	% Right		
Staff nurses	22	74	19	16.5		
3rd year students	34	86	16	11.8	S.N./1	$P < .01$
2nd year students	37	92	14	9.8	3/1	$P < .01$
1st year students	69	57	12	8.7		

TABLE 19

SUMMARY OF SIGNIFICANT DIFFERENCES BETWEEN THE MEAN SCORES OF EACH GROUP OF NURSES IN SCIENCE TEST, COMPARED ON NINETEEN QUESTIONS

+ = the mean score of the more senior group is higher
− = the mean score of the more junior group is higher

Differences highly significant ($p < .01$) unless indicated by *, when $p < .05$

Number of years between groups	Group	Question number																				Totals
		1	2	3	4	5	6	7	8	9	10	11	12	13	14	15	16	17	18	19	
One year's difference	Staff nurses/3rd year students					*+		+										+			4+
	Third year/2nd year students				+								*−							+	2+ 1−
	Second year/1st year students	+		+	+				*+		*+	+	+	*		*+		+	+	+	10+
Two years' difference	Staff nurses/2nd year students	+	+	+	+			+				+	−	*	+	+	+		+	+	8+ 1−
	Third year/1st year students	+	*+	+	+	+	+		*+			+		+	+	+	+	+	+	+	13+
Three years' difference	Staff nurses/1st year students	+	+	+	+	+		+	+			+		+	+	*+	+	+	+	+	13+
For each question	Sum of +	4	3	4	5	4	1	2	1	2	1	5	1	4	3	3	2	4	2	5	50+
	Sum of −												2								2−

4.2.3 Comparison of nurses' scores in the Science Test in items classified according to the sciences: the mean score of each group of nurses compared with the mean score of each of the other groups (Tables 20 to 27, pp. 91-97).

The items in the test were classified according to the science from which they are derived.

In each science subject the differences between the mean score of each group of nurses was tested by analysis of variance. None of the differences were significant.

Table 20 shows the mean score of each group in each science. Although no significant differences were found, it would seem that there is a trend towards higher scores in the more senior groups of nurses.

From the results of these analyses it can be seen that the wide variations which were found between the groups of nurses in relation to whole questions can not be attributed to differences in the levels of knowledge in any of the individual sciences.

TABLE 20

MEAN SCORES OF NURSES IN EACH GROUP IN ITEMS CLASSIFIED
ACCORDING TO THE SCIENCES

Group	Physi-ology	Micro-biology	Path-ology	Pharma-cology	Physics	Chemis-try	Arith-metic
Staff nurses (N = 115)	13.24	16.10	8.66	9.55	4.68	0.79	3.69
3rd year students (N = 136)	12.67	15.44	8.09	8.20	4.43	0.76	3.24
2nd year students (N = 143)	12.76	15.62	7.45	7.99	4.52	0.57	2.36
1st year students (N = 138)	11.40	14.65	4.67	6.21	3.68	0.84	1.47
	N = 24	N = 29	N = 14	N = 13	N = 9	N = 2	N = 7

No significant differences were found between the mean scores
of any group in any of the sciences.

TABLE 21

NURSES' SCORES ON PHYSIOLOGY ITEMS IN THE SCIENCE TEST: RAW DATA
AND MEAN SCORES (N = 24)

Question number	Item number	Activity	Staff nurses (N = 115)	3rd year students (N = 143)	2nd year students (N = 143)	1st year students (N = 138)
				Raw scores		
1	1	Getting a patient up	88	86	104	82
2	5	Surgical dressing technique	31	32	13	44
3	1	Urine testing	63	54	49	24
5	1	Oral hygiene	51	55	44	49
7	1	Abdominal paracentesis	83	53	-	-
8	3	Collection of specimens: microbiological	85	90	95	57
9	1	Pressure areas	34	39	35	16
9	3	Pressure areas	49	60	59	66
9	4	Pressure areas	103	126	128	121
9	5	Pressure areas	49	52	51	46
11	1	Weighing patients	67	59	81	69
12	1	Physiology of blood pressure	89	89	100	100
12	2	Physiology of blood pressure	55	73	82	67
12	3	Physiology of blood pressure	85	104	104	69
12	4	Physiology of blood pressure	62	96	113	103
12	5	Physiology of blood pressure	94	110	131	114
12	6	Physiology of blood pressure	99	119	132	108
13	6	Bladder irrigation	83	95	91	60
15	3	Treatment of eyes	27	26	27	30
18	1	Haemorrhage and pulse rate	99	112	118	79
18	2	Haemorrhage and pulse rate	41	59	54	65
18	3	Haemorrhage and pulse rate	55	66	74	68
18	4	Haemorrhage and pulse rate	37	49	47	42
18	5	Haemorrhage and pulse rate	87	97	92	72

MEAN SCORES

Staff nurses (N = 115)	3rd year students (N = 136)	2nd year students (N = 143)	1st year students (N = 138)
13.24	12.67	12.76	11.40

TABLE 22

NURSES' SCORES ON MICROBIOLOGY ITEMS IN THE TEST:
RAW DATA AND MEAN SCORES (N = 29)

Question number	Item number	Activity	Staff nurses (N = 115)	Raw Scores 3rd year students (N = 136)	2nd year students (N = 143)	1st year students (N = 138)
2	1	Surgical dressing technique	28	41	40	25
2	2	Surgical dressing technique	92	107	111	103
2	3	Surgical dressing technique	42	26	28	20
2	4	Surgical dressing technique	93	98	98	89
2	6	Surgical dressing technique	93	110	112	96
3	5	Urine testing	105	129	112	82
4	3	Preparation for operation	103	123	115	109
6	1	Bathing patients: disinfection of bath	68	82	98	96
6	2	Bathing patients: disinfection of bath	103	113	121	120
6	4	Bathing patients: disinfection of bath	75	76	88	71
6	6	Bathing patients: disinfection of bath	51	57	60	66
7	3	Abdominal paracentesis	87	106	-	-
7	5	Abdominal paracentesis	44	42	-	-
8	1	Collection of specimens: *(microbiological)*	56	73	76	72
8	2	Collection of specimens: *(microbiological)*	62	66	62	54
8	4	Collection of specimens: *(microbiological)*	34	38	38	42
8	5	Collection of specimens: *(microbiological)*	82	90	92	95
8	6	Collection of specimens: *(microbiological)*	76	80	88	76
9	2	Pressure areas	80	114	116	120
10	1	Sterilisation by autoclaving	8	12	14	10
10	3	Sterilisation by autoclaving	56	63	77	63
10	4	Sterilisation by autoclaving	68	86	83	61
10	5	Sterilisation by autoclaving	13	15	22	27
10	6	Sterilisation by autoclaving	76	68	102	69
14	5	Sterilisation by boiling	47	48	54	40
14	6	Sterilisation by boiling	103	121	125	129
15	1	Treatment of eyes	88	116	129	106
15	2	Treatment of eyes	97	109	103	96
15	5	Treatment of eyes	52	70	70	56

Mean Scores

Staff Nurses (N = 115)	3rd year students (N = 136)	2nd year students (N = 143)	1st year students (N = 138)
16.10	15.44	15.62	14.65

TABLE 23

NURSES' SCORES ON PATHOLOGY ITEMS IN THE SCIENCE TEST:
RAW DATA AND MEAN SCORES (N = 14)

Question number	Item number	Activity	Staff nurses (N = 115)	2nd year students (N = 143)	3rd year students (N = 136)	1st year students (N = 138)
				Raw Scores		
1	3	Getting a patient up	88	109	93	97
1	4	Getting a patient up	94	110	101	63
3	2	Urine testing	18	27	32	16
3	4	Urine testing	31	30	24	14
4	1	Preparation for operation	109	124	123	102
4	2	Preparation for operation	113	128	123	101
4	6	Preparation for operation	113	130	133	122
5	2	Oral hygiene	30	28	14	28
5	3	Oral hygiene	60	54	57	46
5	4	Oral hygiene	20	18	18	9
5	5	Oral hygiene	92	95	68	37
11	2	Weighing patients	70	79	99	80
11	6	Weighing patients	89	111	116	104
13	3	Bladder irrigation	69	74	65	41

MEAN SCORES

Staff nurses (N = 115)	3rd year students (N = 136)	2nd year students (N = 143)	1st year students (N = 138)
8.66	8.09	7.45	4.67

TABLE 24

NURSES' SCORES ON PHARMACOLOGY ITEMS IN THE SCIENCE TEST:
RAW DATA AND MEAN SCORES (N = 13)

Question number	Item number	Activity	Raw Scores			
			Staff nurses (N = 115)	3rd year students (N = 136)	2nd year students (N = 143)	1st year students (N = 138)
1	2	Getting a patient up	70	63	60	59
4	4	Preparation for operation	108	127	118	82
4	5	Preparation for operation	110	131	121	90
6	5	Bathing patients: disinfection of bath	22	20	23	29
11	3	Weighing patients	101	101	102	67
11	4	Weighing patients	67	43	19	11
11	5	Weighing patients	98	114	110	89
15	4	Treatment of eyes	86	95	93	81
17	1	Blood concentration of drugs	90	95	103	67
17	2	Blood concentration of drugs	58	45	67	46
17	3	Blood concentration of drugs	103	110	120	83
17	4	Blood concentration of drugs	83	84	92	71
17	5	Blood concentration of drugs	102	110	114	69

MEAN SCORES

Staff nurses (N = 115)	3rd year students (N = 136)	2nd year students (N = 143)	1st year students (N = 138)
9.55	8.2	7.99	6.21

TABLE 25

NURSES' SCORES ON PHYSICS ITEMS IN THE SCIENCE TEST: RAW DATA
AND MEAN SCORES (N = 9)

Question number	Item number	Activity	Raw Scores			
			Staff nurses (N = 115)	3rd year students (N = 136)	2nd year students (N = 143)	1st year students (N = 138)
3	3	Urine testing	64	70	76	62
5	6	Oral hygiene	72	78	99	81
10	2	Sterilisation by autoclaving	37	64	64	62
13	1	Bladder irrigation	63	73	76	27
13	2	Bladder irrigation	53	63	53	35
13	4	Bladder irrigation	74	79	81	59
13	5	Bladder irrigation	50	56	58	52
14	3	Sterilisation by boiling	37	31	31	24
14	4	Sterilisation by boiling	88	97	109	98

MEAN SCORES

Staff nurses (N = 115)	3rd year students (N = 136)	2nd year students (N = 143)	1st year students (N = 138)
4.68	4.43	4.52	3.68

TABLE 26

NURSES' SCORES ON CHEMISTRY ITEMS IN THE SCIENCE TEST:
RAW DATA AND MEAN SCORES (N = 2)

Question number	Item number	Activity	Raw Scores			
			Staff nurses (N = 115)	3rd year students (N = 136)	2nd year students (N = 143)	1st year students (N = 138)
14	1	Sterilisation by boiling	41	42	21	72
14	2	Sterilisation by boiling	50	63	60	42

MEAN SCORES

Staff nurses (N = 115)	3rd year students (N = 136)	2nd year students (N = 143)	1st year students (N = 138)
0.79	0.76	0.57	0.84

TABLE 27

NURSES' SCORES ON ARITHMETIC ITEMS IN THE SCIENCE TEST:
RAW DATA AND MEAN SCORES (N = 7)

Question number	Item number	Activity	Raw Scores			
			Staff nurses (N = 115)	3rd year students (N = 136)	2nd year students (N = 143)	1st year students (N = 138)
16		Regulation of intravenous fluids	19	16	14	12
19	1	Conversion of drug dosages	79	78	64	39
19	2	Conversion of drug dosages	67	78	65	34
19	3	Conversion of drug dosages	78	77	62	31
19	4	Conversion of drug dosages	63	71	48	32
19	5	Conversion of drug dosages	43	45	31	19
19	6	Conversion of drug dosages	75	75	53	36

MEAN SCORES

Staff nurses (N = 115)	3rd year students (N = 136)	2nd year students (N = 143)	1st year students (N = 138)
3.69	3.24	2.36	1.47

4.3 CORRELATION BETWEEN THE NURSES' SCORES IN THE SCIENCE TEST AND THE FREQUENCY WITH WHICH EACH GROUP WAS OBSERVED TO CARRY OUT ACTIVITIES ASSOCIATED WITH THE QUESTIONS (Table 28, p. 99)

Two calculations were carried out using the following data:
a. the scores achieved in each question by each group of nurses, expressed as a percentage of the score possible on each question;
b. the frequency with which each group was observed to carry out the activities associated with each question, expressed as a percentage of the total frequency with which these activities were seen to be carried out.

Spearman rank-difference method of calculating the co-efficients of correlation was used (Garrett, 1958c).

The terminology used in describing these analyses is a modified version of that used by Garrett (1958e);

r from .00 to -.40 denotes indifferent or low correlation
r from -.40 to -.70 denotes substantial or marked relationship
r from -.70 to -1.00 denotes high or very high correlation.

4.3.1 Correlation, for each group of nurses, between their scores on all the questions in the Science Test and the frequency with which they were observed to carry out activities associated with the questions (Table 28, p. 99)

For each group of nurses the rank-differences between these two factors on all the questions were used and the coefficients of correlation found were:

staff nurses	Rho = +.30
third year students	Rho = -.49
second year students	Rho = +.10
first year students	Rho = -.05

Although the staff nurses' correlation is low it is positive. This is the only group where there is some relationship between their level of knowledge of the biological sciences and the activities which they perform. The higher negative correlation demonstrated in the third year student group may result from the fact that this group is expected to act in almost a staff nurse capacity before having passed the final state examination. It may be that it is in their studies in preparation for this examination that they bridge the gap between their knowledge and that of the staff nurses. Over the 18 questions the correlations between the scores and the frequency of observation in the first and second year students are too low to indicate any relationship between the two factors.

TABLE 28

CORRELATION BETWEEN NURSES' SCORES IN SCIENCE TEST AND THE FREQUENCY OF OBSERVATION
OF ACTIVITIES ASSOCIATED WITH THE TEST QUESTIONS

Question number	Activity	Staff nurses (N = 115)		3rd year students (N = 136)		2nd year students (N = 143)		1st year students (N = 138)		Coefficient of correlation Rho
		Scores %	Obs. %	Scores %	Obs. %	Scores %	Obs. %	Scores %	Obs. %	
1	Getting a patient up	73.9	24.0	67.6	11.5	62.6	23.0	54.5	41.5	- .4
2	Surgical dressing technique	54.9	24.6	50.7	34.4	46.9	18.8	45.5	22.1	+ .6
3	Urine testing	49.0	10.8	45.6	25.8	41.0	22.1	28.7	41.3	- .8
4	Preparation for operation	95.1	38.1	93.5	20.4	86.1	21.8	73.2	19.7	+ .8
5	Oral hygiene	47.1	2.9	40.2	7.5	34.8	20.8	30.2	68.7	-1.0
6	Bathing patients: disinfection of bath	66.8	12.5	63.2	7.9	68.1	24.8	67.8	54.8	+ .8
7	Abdominal paracentesis	64.9	72.4	57.1	27.6	-	-	-	-	+1.0
8	Collection of specimens: (microbiological)	57.2	13.9	53.6	22.1	52.6	13.9	47.8	50.0	- .6
9	Pressure areas	54.8	8.8	57.5	18.3	54.4	22.5	53.5	50.5	- .8
10	Sterilisation by autoclaving	37.4	41.1	37.7	20.6	42.2	11.9	35.3	26.4	- .8
11	Weighing patients	71.6	72.2	62.1	2.9	61.4	8.9	50.6	15.9	+ .2
12	Physiology of blood pressure	70.1	20.0	72.4	24.1	77.2	26.5	67.8	29.3	- .2
13	Bladder irrigation	56.5	20.3	53.9	25.8	49.4	29.7	33.0	24.2	- .4
14	Sterilisation by boiling	53.0	20.0	49.3	33.3	46.7	30.4	48.9	16.3	0
15	Treatment of eyes	60.7	23.8	61.2	28.7	59.0	31.5	53.5	16.1	+ .4
16	Regulation of Intraveneous fluids	16.5	25.1	11.8	33.7	9.8	22.4	8.7	18.9	+ .8
17	Blood concentration of drugs	75.8	32.9	65.4	31.7	69.5	18.2	48.7	17.1	+ .8
18	Haemorrhage and pulse rate	55.7	9.4	56.5	20.7	53.4	25.3	47.2	44.6	- .8
19	Conversion of drug dosages	58.8	33.2	52.0	31.3	37.6	18.1	23.1	17.5	+1.0
		Rho = + .30		Rho = - .49		Rho = + .10		Rho = - .05		

4.3.2 Correlation, for each question in the Science Test, between the score of each group of nurses and the frequency with which each group was observed to carry out activities associated with the questions (Table 28)

It will be seen from Table 28 that there was a substantial or high positive correlation in seven questions, negative correlation to a similar degree in six questions, and low or negligible correlation in six questions.

Table 29 shows the questions in which there was a substantial or high positive correlation.

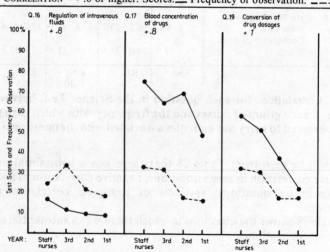

FIGURE 9a (SEE TABLE 29)

CORRELATION BETWEEN NURSES' SCORES IN SCIENCE TEST AND
FREQUENCY WITH WHICH ACTIVITIES WERE OBSERVED TO BE CARRIED OUT:

CORRELATION = +.6 OR HIGHER. Scores:_____ Frequency of observation:_ _ _ _

FIGURE 9a CONTINUED (TABLE 29)

CORRELATION BETWEEN NURSES' SCORES IN SCIENCE TEST AND FREQUENCY
WITH WHICH ACTIVITIES WERE OBSERVED TO BE CARRIED OUT:

CORRELATION = + .6 or higher. Scores:___ Frequency of observation: _ _ _ _

TABLE 29

QUESTIONS IN THE SCIENCE TEST IN WHICH
CORRELATIONS WERE + .5 OR HIGHER

Question number	Activity	Coefficient of correlation Rho
2	Surgical dressing technique	+.6
6	Bathing patients: disinfection of bath	+.8
7	Abdominal paracentesis	+ 1
16	Regulation of intravenous fluids	+.8
17	Blood concentration of drugs	+.8
19	Conversion of drug dosages	+ 1

In relation to the correlations shown in Table 29 it is apparent that the groups of nurses carrying out the activities are those who have most knowledge of the biological sciences upon which the activities depend. With the exception of *question* 6, staff nurses and third year students joinly carried out the activities more frequently than did the second and first year students together. The junior groups not only carried out the activities associated with question 6 more frequently, but showed that they had more knowledge of the microbiology and pharmacology involved in disinfection although the differences in scores were not significant.

In *question* 16, although the correlation coefficient was +.8, it is notable that the scores in this question were low for all groups of nurses. It would seem from this that it is not customary for nursing staff, when regulating the flow of intravenous fluids, to think in terms of drops per minute. If the fluid flow is regulated according to the large scale of measurement commonly used in the doctors' prescription, for example, 500 ml in 4 hours, the only way that this could be done would be by simply looking at the apparatus and adjusting the rate of flow to what 'looks right'. The degree of accuracy likely to be achieved by this method would not be accepted in relation to the administration of a drug by any other route.

Table 30 shows the questions in which there was a substantial or high negative correlation.

From Table 28 it can be seen that the groups of nurses with the highest scores in these questions are not the groups who most frequently carry out the activities associated with the questions.

With the exception of *question* 10, first and second year students jointly carried out the activities associated with these questions more frequently than did third year students and staff nurses together. In this question, staff nurses and first year students jointly carried out the associated activities more frequently, while third and second year students showed that they had more knowledge of the physics and microbiology involved in sterilising by the use of steam under pressure. However, the only significant difference between scores was between second and first year students.

In the remaining questions in this group the first year students were seen to carry out the associated activities with considerably higher frequency than the other groups and an inspection of the scores of the groups in these questions reveals that, with the exception of *question* 9, first year students had considerably lower scores than did the other groups.

It appears that the more senior nurses on duty who decide who shall give what nursing care often do this without regard for the knowledge and understanding of the activity possessed by the person to whom the work is assigned. In such circumstances it would seem that the more junior students are expected to function on a mechanical level. They are told what to do and, as long as they appear to know how to carry out the activity, this is all that is required of them.

Some of these activities, such as urine testing and autoclaving, do not necessitate direct contact with the patients. These procedures could be satisfactorily carried out by a technician who need never see a patient. As regards the other activities in this group, for example, oral hygiene, care of pressure areas and taking the pulse, the students must necessarily be in close personal contact with patients. In these cases the performance of the activity carries with it the responsibility to observe the patient's condition and his response to the treatment. With the limited knowledge of the appropriate biological sciences which the first year students have demonstrated, it is doubtful whether they can be expected to recognise changes, or the significance of changes, in the patient's condition and to report these to the nurse in charge of the ward.

If this is the level at which a considerable proportion of nursing care can effectively be carried out, it would seem that student nurses are not required for this purpose. At such a level, the work could be done as well by a nursing auxiliary who had had the necessary in-service training, and probably better by an enrolled nurse.

It is clear from these data that the junior students fulfill a service function in the wards and that their knowledge of the biological sciences upon which an understanding of an activity depends is not enhanced by repeatedly performing the activity.

FIGURE 9b (SEE TABLE 30)

CORRELATION BETWEEN NURSES' SCORES IN SCIENCE TEST AND FREQUENCY WITH WHICH ACTIVITIES WERE OBSERVED TO BE CARRIED OUT:

CORRELATION = -.6 OR HIGHER. Scores: _____   Frequency of observation: -----

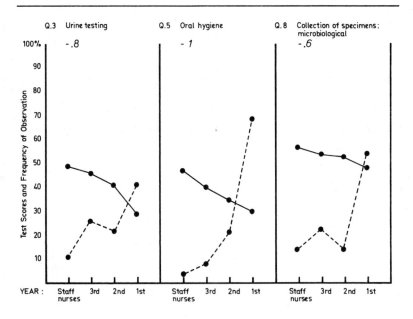

FIGURE 9b CONTINUED (TABLE 30)

CORRELATIONBETWEEN NURSES' SCORES IN SCIENCE TEST AND FREQUENCY WITH
WHICH ACTIVITIES WERE OBSERVED TO BE CARRIED OUT:

CORRELATION = -.6 or higher. Scores:_____ Frequency of observation:_ _ _

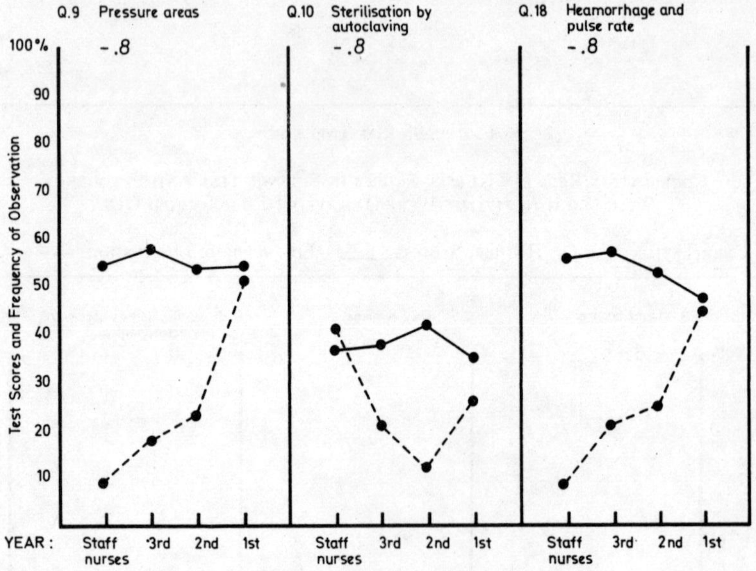

TABLE 30

QUESTIONS IN THE SCIENCE TEST IN WHICH CORRELATIONS
WERE -.5 OR HIGHER

Question number	Activity	Coefficient of correlation Rho
3	Urine testing	-.8
5	Oral hygiene	- 1
8	Collection of specimens: microbiological	-.6
9	Pressure areas	-.8
10	Autoclaving	-.8
18	Haemorrhage and pulse rate	-.8

In the remaining six questions the coefficients of correlation were indifferent or low.

TABLE 31

QUESTIONS IN THE SCIENCE TEST IN WHICH CORRELATIONS
WERE LESS THAN ±.5

Question number	Activity	Coefficient of correlation Rho
1	Getting a patient up	-.4
11	Weighing patients	+.2
12	Physiology of blood pressure	+.2
13	Bladder irrigation	-.4
14	Sterilisation by boiling	0
15	Treatment of patients' eyes	+.4

As it would be expected from Table 31, within this group of correlations no pattern emerges in relation to the scores of the different groups of nurses and the frequency with which they were observed to carry out the activities associated with the questions.

4.4 DISCUSSION OF THE FINDINGS

Although some entrants to nursing may have some knowledge of the biological sciences, and further knowledge may be acquired after completing training, staff nurses are the finished products of a three-year basic nursing education and their knowledge is derived mainly from their learning during this period. If there is a progressive acquisition of knowledge throughout the three year training programme, it could be expected that the scores of the students and staff nurses on the Science Test would follow the same pattern, that is, become higher with each successive year.

This is supported by the findings of this study when the mean scores of the groups in the whole Science Test are compared. However, when considering the differences between the scores of the four groups in the individual questions, this consistent pattern is to be seen only between first and second year students.

In the present study a considerable amount of learning was found to take place towards the end of the first year and at the beginning of the second year. This may be associated with the fact that when these data were collected there was a Preliminary State Examination taken at the end of the first year of training which included a paper on anatomy, physiology, health and nutrition. This was the only statutory examination in which there was a paper allotted exclusively to the biological sciences. Having passed the Preliminary State Examination the students may have felt that there was no need to give further attention to the biological science content in their later studies.

Very few differences were found between the scores of staff nurses and third year students and between those of third and second year students. There was no consistency in the pattern of questions in which differences occurred. The questions where there were differences between staff nurses and third year students were not the same as those where there were differences between third and second year students.

In about one third of the activities about which questions were asked, the groups of nurses with most knowledge of the biological sciences upon which the activities depend were seen to carry out the activities. In the remaining two thirds, the groups carried out either the activities about which they had least knowledge or there was no meaningful relationship between knowledge and frequency of observation.

These findings would seem to support the idea that the student/employee status of the student nurse is unsatisfactory, at least in relation to first and second year students. They also raise questions about the quality of care which is provided for patients in hospital. Sexton (1970) suggested that patients may not be aware that much of their nursing care is given by students.

Third year students could be viewed somewhat differently. There were differences between the scores of third year students and staff nurses in only four questions, and the frequency with which activities were carried out by the third year students followed a pattern more similar to that of staff nurses than to those of the other two groups. It would seem from this that students in their third year of training commonly act in the capacity of staff nurses.

The fact that the differences between these two groups are so slight raises the question of whether all students need wait for three years before taking the written part of the Final State Examination, at least in so far as it depends upon a knowledge of the biological sciences.

5. Findings: Nurses' I.Qs. and Educational Attainment

5.1 INTRODUCTION

The problem of selecting 'suitable' candidates for nursing has been recognised for a long time as one of considerable complexity.

Some of the factors involved are known to be personality, intelligence, general educational attainment and interest in nursing.

From the literature reviewed in the introduction to this study it is evident that the conditions under which student nurses work are such that they must take a considerable amount of the responsibility for their own learning. Although all the factors mentioned above are likely to influence the ability of students to study on their own, only I.Qs. and general educational attainment are included in the present study.

In this section the relationships which were found between these two factors and the scores achieved by the nurses in the Science Test will be described.

The coefficients of correlation between the Science Test scores and school attainment, and between the Science Test scores and intelligence quotients were calculated for each group of nurses using the product-moment method of computing r when deviations are taken from zero (Garrett, 1958d).

Some respondents had passed in subjects in the Scottish Certificate of Education (S.C.E.) and some in the General Certificate of Education (G.C.E.) examinations. Higher grade passes in the S.C.E. and Advanced level passes in the G.C.E. examinations were grouped together for the purposes of statistical analyses and will be referred to in the text and in the tables as higher passes. Ordinary level passes in the G.C.E. and in the S.C.E. examinations after 1962 and Lower grade passes before that date were grouped together and will be referred to as ordinary passes. In the second group, respondents who had passes in any subjects at higher level were excluded.

5.2 CORRELATION, FOR EACH GROUP OF NURSES, BETWEEN THE SCORES IN THE SCIENCE TEST AND THE NUMBER OF PASSES IN SCHOOL EXAMINATION SUBJECTS
(Table 32 p. 109; Table 33, p. 110)

It was found that there was a wide range of educational attainment within the sample of nurses. The distribution of passes in school subjects over the four groups together (N = 532) was as follows:

23.98 per cent   no school certificate passes;
42.67 per cent   passes in at least one subject at ordinary level;
33.44 per cent   passes in at least one subject at higher level.

For each group of nurses eight correlations were calculated using scores on the Science Test and the number of passes in school examination subjects.

The following correlations were calculated between nurses' scores in the Science Test and the number of passes in school examination subjects at higher level (Table 32, p. 109):

a. passes at higher level in any subject and the scores of all the members of a group (Table 32, column a);
b. passes at higher level in any subject and the scores of those members of a group who had passes at higher level (Table 32, column b);
c. passes at higher level in science subjects and the scores of all the members of a group (Table 32, column c);
d. passes at higher level in science subjects and the scores of those members of a group who had passes at higher level in science subjects (Table 32, column d).

The following correlations were calculated between nurses' scores in the Science Test and the number of passes in school examination subjects at ordinary level (Table 33, p. 110):

a. passes at ordinary level in any subject and the scores of all the members of a group (Table 33, column a);
b. passes at ordinary level in any subject and the scores of those members of a group who had passes at ordinary level (Table 33, column b);
c. passes at ordinary level in science subjects and the scores of all the members of a group (Table 33, column c);
d. passes at ordinary level in science subjects and the scores of those members of a group who had passes at ordinary level in science subjects (Table 33, column d).

Table 34 shows the number of nurses in each group who had passes at higher and ordinary levels and the subdivision of these figures to show the number who had passes in science subjects at these two levels.

It will be seen from Table 34 that less than half of the people with passes at higher level had passes in science subjects. Because of this small number, the correlations shown in columns (c) and (d) in Table 32 should be viewed with some reservations. In columns (a) and (b) of Table 32 it will be seen that all the correlations are positive although only in the third year student group was there a substantial relationship between the number of passes at higher level and the scores in the Science Test of those with passes at this level (r = +.56).

Table 34 shows that in each group of nurses there was a greater number of people with passes at ordinary level. In the staff nurse, third year student and second year student groups more than 80 per cent of those with ordinary level passes had passes in science subjects. In the first year group the percentage was 75.5.

In Table 33 it will be seen that the correlations between the ordinary level passes and the scores obtained in the Science Test were very variable and that with one exception the relationship between the factors was indifferent or low. The exception was the high positive correlation (r = +.84) between the number of passes at ordinary level in science subjects and the scores of those with passes at this level in science subjects in the first year student group (Table 33, column b).

TABLE 32

CORRELATION, FOR EACH GROUP OF NURSES, BETWEEN THE NUMBER WITH PASSES IN SCHOOL SUBJECTS AT HIGHER LEVEL AND SCORES IN THE SCIENCE TEST

Figures in brackets; the first denotes the number with higher passes in each group; the second denotes:-
columns (a) and (c): the total number of nurses in each group;
columns (b) and (d): the number of nurses in each group with passes at higher level.

Group	a Number with higher level passes/scores of whole group	b Number with higher level passes/ scores of those with higher passes	c Number with higher level passes in sciences/scores of whole group	d Number with higher level passes in sciences/scores of those with higher passes in sciences
Staff nurses (N = 115)	+ .31 (36:115)	+ .43 (36:36)	+ .06 (16:115)	+ .18 (16:16)
3rd year students (N = 136)	+ .29 (42:136)	+ .56 (42:42)	+ .22 (20:136)	+ .67 (20:20)
2nd year students (N = 143)	+ .25 (45:143)	+ .49 (45:45)	+ .11 (19:143)	- .05 (19:19)
1st year students (N = 138)	+ .48 (55:138)	+ .38 (55:55)	+ .32 (17:138)	+ .43 (17:17)

TABLE 33

CORRELATION, FOR EACH GROUP OF NURSES, BETWEEN THE NUMBER WITH PASSES IN
SCHOOL SUBJECTS AT ORDINARY LEVEL AND SCORES IN THE SCIENCE TEST

Figures in brackets: the first denotes the number with ordinary passes in each group: the
second denotes:-
columns (a) and (c): the total number of nurses in each group;
columns (b) and (d): the number of nurses in each group with passes at ordinary level.

Group	a Number with ordinary level passes/scores of whole group	b Number with ordinary level passes/scores of those with ordinary passes	c Number with level passes in sciences/scores of whole group	d Number with ordinary level passes in sciences/ scores of those with ordinary passes in sciences
Staff nurses (N = 115)	- .07 (49:115)	+ .24 (49:49)	- .15 (40:115)	+ .05 (40:40)
3rd year students (N = 136)	+ .13 (51:136)	+ .38 (51:51)	+ .08 (44:136)	+ .31 (44:44)
2nd year students (N = 143)	+ .32 (70:143)	+ .36 (70:70)	+ .31 (58:143)	+ .23 (58:58)
1st year students (N = 138)	- .04 (57:138)	+ .84 (57:57)	- .16 (43:138)	+ .14 (43:43)

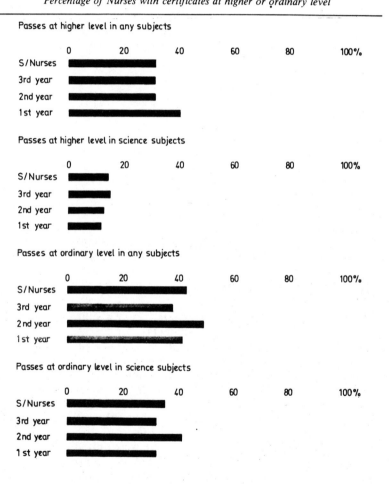

FIGURE 10 (SEE TABLE 34)

EDUCATIONAL QUALIFICATIONS OF EACH GROUP OF NURSES

Percentage of Nurses with certificates at higher or ordinary level

Passes at higher level in any subjects

Passes at higher level in science subjects

Passes at ordinary level in any subjects

Passes at ordinary level in science subjects

TABLE 34

PERCENTAGE OF NURSES IN EACH GROUP WITH PASSES IN SCHOOL CERTIFICATE SUBJECTS;
RAW FIGURES IN BRACKETS

Group	a Passes at higher level in any subject %	b Passes at higher level in a science subject %	c Passes at ordinary level in any subject %	d Passes at ordinary level in a science subject %
Staff nurses (N = 115)	31.31 (36)	13.91 (16)	42.52 (49)	34.78 (40)
3rd year students (N = 136)	30.88 (42)	14.71 (20)	38.14 (51)	32.35 (44)
2nd year students (N = 143)	31.47 (45)	13.29 (19)	48.95 (70)	40.56 (58)
1st year students (N = 138)	39.56 (55)	12.32 (17)	41.32 (57)	31.60 (43)

5.3 CORRELATION, FOR EACH GROUP OF NURSES, BETWEEN SCORES IN THE SCIENCE TEST AND I.Qs.

The correlations found from these calculations were:

staff nurses	$r = +.55$
third year students	$r = +.40$
second year students	$r = +.39$
first year students	$r = +.40$

Within the student groups there was notable consistency in these correlations. Although the levels of correlation must be considered to be moderate, they are just below the line drawn somewhat arbitrarily between a low and a substantial relationship between two factors. Within the staff nurse group, there was a substantial relationship between scores in the Science Test and I.Qs.

From Table 35 it will be seen that there were only slight differences between the mean I.Qs. of the four groups of nurses, none of which was significant. It will also be seen that there was a high percentage of nurses at the upper end of the I.Q. scale. This was most marked in the staff nurse and first year student groups. The third year group was the only one in which the majority of its members did not have an I.Q. of 111 or higher.

FIGURE 11 (SEE TABLE 35)

DISTRIBUTION OF INTELLIGENCE QUOTIENTS AMONG THE
TOTAL SAMPLE OF NURSES (N = 532)

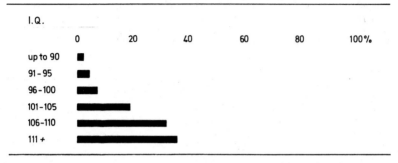

TABLE 35

THE RANGE AND DISTRIBUTION OF THE I.Qs. WITHIN THE FOUR GROUPS OF NURSES
AND THE MEAN I.Q. FOR EACH GROUP

I.Q.	Staff nurses N = 115 %	3rd year students N = 136 %	2nd year students N = 143 %	1st year students N = 138 %	Total N = 532 %
up to 90	1.74	0.74	0.70	2.90	1.50
91 - 95	2.60	5.88	2.80	4.35	3.95
96 - 100	6.96	5.15	8.39	8.70	7.33
101 - 105	23.48	23.53	15.38	13.77	18.80
106 - 110	25.22	41.18	34.27	27.54	32.33
111 +	40.0	23.53	38.46	42.75	36.09
Mean I.Q.	110.1	108.9	110.1	109.1	109.7

Table 36 shows that there was a remarkable similarity between the four groups of nurses in relation to the mean I.Q. and the mean number of passes in school subjects at higher and ordinary levels. When compared by analysis of variance none of the differences between the groups was found to be significant. It is interesting, however, that the differences between the mean scores achieved by each group in the Science Test were found to be highly significant.

TABLE 36

FOR EACH GROUP OF NURSES:

Column (a)   MEAN I.Q. SCORED ON OTIS INTERMEDIATE TEST
Column (b)   MEAN NUMBER OF PASSES IN SCHOOL SUBJECTS AT HIGHER LEVEL
Column (c)   MEAN NUMBER OF PASSES IN SCHOOL SUBJECTS AT ORDINARY LEVEL,
                  EXCLUDING THOSE WITH PASSES AT HIGHER LEVEL
Column (d)   MEAN SCORES IN THE SCIENCE TEST

Group	(a) Mean I.Q.	(b) Mean number of higher level passes	(c) Mean number of ordinary level passes	(d) Mean scores on science test
Staff nurses (N = 115)	110.1	0.76	1.79	60.03
3rd year students (N = 136)	108.9	0.71	1.48	56.43
2nd year students (N = 143)	110.1	0.66	1.92	51.79
1st year students (N = 138)	109.7	0.82	1.63	43.94

Columns (a), (b) and (c): no significant differences between means for each group of nurses
Column (d): all differences highly significant ($p < .01$)

5.4 DISCUSSION OF THE FINDINGS

From these results it would seem that the level of intelligence of nurses has had a more consistent effect on their scores in the Science Test than has the level of attainment in school subjects. This finding is in agreement with those reported by MacGuire (1969).

Although school attainment shows little consistency or significance in its effect on the scores in the Science Test it should not be discarded as a means of selecting entrants to nursing. Such a conclusion could be reached only after more detailed study involving a larger sample of nurses with passes at higher level in school subjects, and a variety of tests involving different aspects of nursing. It is possible that a considerable number of those with low educational attainment could have studied to a more advanced level if this had been necessary to gain acceptance as a student nurse. Lancaster (1971) in discussing this subject said:

... it is not known how many people who make up their minds to nurse while still at school are in fact capable of reaching a higher level of education, but make no effort to acquire more than the minimum need for nursing simply because it is not asked for. The only incentive to do so, apart from personal interest, would seem to be a desire to train in a school of nursing which demands a higher standard.

Although the present study was only concerned with nurses' knowledge of the biological sciences, these constitute a relatively large proportion of the theory which a nurse is required to learn. It might be expected that the level of knowledge of biological sciences related to nursing would depend more on academic ability measurable in terms of school attainment, particularly in science subjects, than would the practical nursing skills on which so much emphasis seems to be placed by both nurses and doctors. Yet analysis of the results has shown only a small degree of correlation between the nurses' school attainment and their Science Test scores.

While the minimum educational standard required for entry to nursing remains low, the number of certificates obtained at school would appear to be an unreliable guide to a nurse's academic ability. Nurses with a few certificates, or with certificates at a low level, may be just as intellectually able as nurses with more certificates, or with certificates at a higher level. A number of other factors contribute to achievement at school, to choice of career and, in the case of nursing, to choice of training school.

In such a situation, it may be that intelligence testing would be a more reliable measure to be used in the selection of students until more information is available about the effects of school attainment.

6. Conclusions and Discussion

6.1 SUMMARY OF FINDINGS

6.1.1 Data obtained from staff nurses' Science Test and Doctors' Questionnaire

a. The staff nurses' knowledge of the biological sciences, represented by their scores in 11 questions in the Science Test, was compared with the doctors' expectations of the staff nurses' knowledge. In eight questions the doctors' expectations were significantly greater than the knowledge displayed by the nurses; in two questions the staff nurses' scores were higher than the doctors expected; in one question there was no significant difference.

b. In eight questions, doctors were asked whether they would prescribe specific treatments in detail, or whether they would expect staff nurses to initiate, carry out and take responsibility for these procedures without detailed instructions. With the exception of one question (on the treatment of eyes) more than half the doctors said that they would expect nurses to carry out treatment without detailed prescription.

c. When the question items were classified according to the different biological sciences, no differences were found between the doctors' expectations and the staff nurses' scores.

d. Doctors' expectations of staff nurses' knowledge did not appear, on the whole, to vary according to the grade of doctor. There were significant differences between the responses of consultants, registrars and house officers in different questions in relation to different nursing activities, but these differences did not conform to any consistent pattern.

e. Doctors were found to have higher expectations of the staff nurses' knowledge when they were provided with the 'correct' answers to the items which comprised the nurses' questions, than when the questions were presented to them in a more general form and related only to the activities on which the questions were based.

6.1.2 Data obtained from staff and student nurses: scores in the Science Test, their I.Q. scores and general educational attainment

a. In the Science Test as a whole it was found that there was a highly significant increase in the mean scores of the groups of nurses with each year of seniority.

b. In the individual questions, the mean scores of the different groups were compared with each other. Of the groups between which there was only one year of seniority, the greatest number of differences was found between the students in the first and second years. There were significant differences between the mean scores of these two groups in ten questions. Between staff nurses and third year students there were differences in four questions, and between third and second year students differences in only two questions. In three questions there were no significant differences between the mean scores of any of the groups.

c. When the question items were classified according to the different biological sciences, no differences were found between the mean scores of the four groups of nurses in any of the sciences.

d. Coefficients of correlation between the scores obtained by each group of nurses, in the Science Test as a whole, and the frequency with which each group was observed to carry out the associated activities, ranged from +.30 for staff nurses to -.49 for third year students. In the second and first year groups the correlations were insignificant.

e. Coefficients of correlation between the scores obtained by each group of nurses, in each of the questions in the Science Test, and the frequency with which each group was observed to carry out the activities associated with each question, ranged from +1 to -1. Of the eighteen questions which were presented to all the groups, the correlation coefficients in six questions were +.50 or higher; in six questions -.50 or higher; in the remaining six they were ±.49 or lower.

f. The mean I.Q. for the whole sample of nurses was 109.55, using the Otis Self-Administering Test of Mental Ability, Intermediate Examination. There was no significant difference between the mean I.Q. scores of the four groups.

g. Of the total sample of nurses (532), 36.09 per cent had I.Q. scores of 111 or over, and 60 per cent had I.Q. scores of 106 or over. In each group of nurses the range extended from below 90 to 116 which is the top of the scale in the Otis Test used.

h. Correlation between the total scores in the Science Test of each group of nurses and their I.Qs. was highest among the staff nurses (+.55). In the three student groups the level was almost constant at +.40; the second year group was marginally lower at +.39.

i. There was no consistent correlation between the nurses' scores in the Science Test and their general educational attainment. The highest positive correlations were between passes at higher level in any subject and the scores of nurses with passes at this level; a substantial relationship (higher than +.4) between these two factors was found in each group except first year students.

The number of nurses who had passes at higher level in science subjects was too small for inferences to be drawn from the correlations.

Correlations between passes at ordinary level and scores on the Science Test were very varied. The only high correlation (+.84) was in the first year group, between the number of passes in any subject and the Science Test scores.

6.2 DISCUSSION OF FINDINGS

6.2.1 Some implications; the case for change

The fact that the staff nurses did not show as much knowledge of the biological sciences related to nursing activities as the doctors expected would seem to have practical implications.

In the hospital situation, where doctors and nurses work in close association in order to provide effective patient care, the discrepancies revealed by these results could be of danger to the patients. Situations could arise in which doctors mistakenly assume that staff nurses understand the aims of the treatments which they prescribe and that the nurses will be able to recognise and report significant changes in the patients' condition.

If the two professions or the public knew of this situation, it seems unlikely that they would be content to allow it to continue.

Two steps could be taken to bridge this gap: either the doctors could modify their expectations, or the level of the staff nurses' knowledge could be raised.

It seems improbable that doctors would be prepared to accept the modifications in the organisation and practice of medicine which would be necessary in order to supervise more closely the care of patients in hospital wards. At the purely practical level, it would mean that they would have to spend a considerably greater part of their time in the wards. This would necessitate an increase in the number of doctors, an increase in the educational facilities, and possibly changes in the medical curriculum.

From the comments in medical journals which were discussed in the introduction, it seems likely that doctors would consider such changes to be a retrograde step. A number of the comments cited indicate that some doctors feel that they are already under severe pressure and that nurses could relieve them of some of their work. For example, it has been suggested by some doctors that district nurses should pay first visits to patients in their homes, that midwives should suture the perineum, that nurses in hospital wards should recognise and initiate treatment for cardiac arrest and that nurses should take more responsibility for patients in intensive care units where complex monitoring machinery is in use.

A decision to raise the standard of the staff nurses' knowledge of the biological sciences related to nursing would have implications for the basic programme of nursing education.

It would not be justifiable to assume that results similar to those of the present study would be found if studies were made of other areas of nursing knowledge using the same methodology. On the other hand it would seem that, if certain changes based on the present findings were made in the organisation of nursing education, such changes could be of some benefit to students' learning in both the biological and social sciences and in the areas of nursing to which they apply.

Staff nurses have already completed their basic programme and have passed the General Nursing Council's examination leading to registration. In order to raise the level of knowledge of the biological sciences it would seem that the General Nursing Council's examination standard would have to be raised. This presents certain difficulties because the panel of examiners is made up of a large number of teachers of nurses, and objective criteria in relation to the standard of knowledge cannot be applied to the essay type of question used. It would seem, therefore, that one method of raising the examination standard would be to use the objective type of question for at least part of the examination. In this way the General Nursing Council would have more direct control of standards and would be less dependent upon the subjective and varied opinions of the panel of examiners.

According to the views of the writers which were quoted and discussed in the introduction, a number of environmental factors are detrimental to the student nurses' learning. Although these writers appeared to be referring to the nurses' learning as a whole, the fact that the biological sciences constitute a large part of that learning makes it reasonable to suppose that their comments include the part of nursing knowledge which is dependent on these sciences. Some of the factors mentioned were the difficulties inherent in the student/employee status of nurses in training, lack of coordination between the theory and practice of nursing, and the deficiencies in the teaching provided in the clinical situation.

It would seem that all these factors are interdependent. Practice in the wards, as far as learning by practising is concerned, is a euphemism for giving any kind of nursing care which the patients may require. In the present study, it was noticed that little attempt seemed to be made to assign nursing activities to students according to the stage of their training. During the period of observation in the wards, the only activities seen to be carried out exclusively by third year students and staff nurses were those which involved assisting doctors with diagnostic tests or treatment, for example, abdominal paracentesis, lumbar puncture, chest aspiration, sternal marrow puncture. All other activities were carried out by first, second and third year students, as well as by staff nurses.

In the present study no attempt was made to evaluate the efficiency with which nursing treatments were performed. It may be that frequent repetition of an activity contributed to the students' technical competence but, if so, this did not appear to affect the level of their knowledge of the related biological sciences.

It would seem that, although some teaching is carried out in the clinical situation, many ward sisters do not have time to teach and the students do not have time to learn. This is hardly surprising if it is accepted that the primary responsibility of the ward sister is to provide for the immediate nursing care of the patients in her charge and that students give a large proportion of this nursing care.

Clinical instructors provide some ward teaching but, as was mentioned previously, they are so few in number that their contribution is inevitably limited.

Since these data were collected there have been some statutory changes in the programme provided for student nurses but the programme as a whole has remained the same length. The minimum time allocated to classroom work has been increased from 24 to 27 weeks, and the theoretical and practical content of the programme is now more broadly based. The work of students is no longer confined to medical and surgical nursing but includes psychiatric, paediatric, obstetric and community nursing.

It would seem that such a programme should produce nurses who could, with more justification, be called general nurses. However, it does not appear to be very realistic to assume that the theoretical study related to the four additional clinical areas could be covered in the three weeks added to the time allocated to classroom work. It would seem more likely that the theoretical content of the medical and surgical nursing part of the programme would be reduced.

At the same time as these changes were being made, the Preliminary State Examination, taken at the end of the first year of training, was discontinued. The effect of this on the nurses' knowledge of the biological sciences is not known. In the present study it was found that there was a considerable difference between the knowledge of first and second year students. It was suggested in paragraph 4.4 that the incentive to study for the Preliminary State Examination, containing a paper on anatomy and physiology, may have been one of the explanations for this difference. This suggestion would seem to be supported by the fact that similar differences were not found between second and third year students.

Although there have been changes in the programme, the status of the student remains the same. From the point of view of the students' employers, the Boards of Management, students spend less time in 'general' medical and surgical wards where previously they could be relied upon to provide relatively long periods of nursing service. It would seem, therefore, that even from a financial point of view, students are of less value to their employers now than they were in the past. During the short time which they spend on secondment to specialist wards and hospitals their services are likely to be of limited value. In some situations students could be more of a liability than an asset.

6.2.2 Suggested changes in the organisation of the basic nursing programme

It would appear that, if the standard of nursing education is to be improved, students need to be provided with an environment in which their opportunities to learn are given the highest priority. A prerequisite of student status for nurses would be the recruitment of other nursing personnel in order to ensure that the hospital services to the community as a whole did not break down. Some steps in this direction have been taken by increasing the numbers of enrolled nurses and part-time registered nurses employed in the hospitals.

If student nurses were not regarded as nursing service personnel, a programme could be arranged in which there was a more effective integration of the practice of nursing and the theory upon which it depends. The present 27 weeks of theoretical study, which are split up into four or six week periods, would seem to be inadequate for students to acquire the knowledge of the biological sciences and other theory upon which nursing depends.

If the teaching staff were free to organise the students' programme without consideration of the service needs of the hospitals, there could be a less rigid division between classroom study and ward practice. It is acknowledged that students must learn the practice of nursing in the clinical situation, and in so doing give nursing service to the hospital. However, in a programme where nursing education had priority the activities carried out by students could be controlled. In the present study it was found that only one third of the nursing activities were carried out by the nurses who had most knowledge of the related biological sciences. It is to be hoped that if clinical practice became an integral part of the nursing education programme, similar results would not be found in the future.

It is suggested that the early part of the nurses' training should be spent in theoretical study; this could be an entirely pre-clinical period, or be associated with nursing practice carried out under carefully controlled conditions. Toward the latter part of their training, they could spend longer periods in the wards to enable them to become an integral part of the nursing team. This should be a progressive process. They could at first be assigned to a patient who required the type of nursing care which they needed to practise. Later, they could spend more time in the ward, giving care to several patients and, towards the end of the programme, assume the responsibilities of full team membership.

This gradual transition, from being a student in the early stages to being a team member towards the end of the programme, would provide students with an opportunity to experience the change of role from student to staff member before having to accept the full responsibilities of the registered nurse. As team members they would also have the opportunity to practise the organisation of patient care for a number of patients and the teaching of more junior students.

However the students' practical experience is arranged, it would seem that students should be provided with the opportunity to become technically proficient at an early stage in the practical part of their programme. They are very conscious of the fact that incompetence and lack of dexterity in carrying out nursing treatments constitute a risk to the patients, or may at least cause them unnecessary discomfort. This can produce considerable anxiety in the students and possibly result in their concentrating on acquiring practical nursing skills to the exclusion of other learning. If they were provided with facilities to practise nursing procedures under supervision until they felt confident in their ability to perform competently, they would then be able to give thought to the patients' needs as a whole, using their knowledge of the biological and other sciences to make decisions about the care which patients require, and about the way in which it could best be organised.

In order to acquire skill by practising nursing, students must inevitably give service to the patients. Nursing service administrators should consider the nursing care given by students in the early part of their training as a welcome addition to the service provided by the hospital. In the later stages of the students' programme, when they are moving into full membership of the nursing team, the contribution which they make to nursing service could be recognised by providing them with remuneration additional to their student grants.

6.2.3 Student nurses' abilities

A reorganisation of the students' curriculum and educational environment would not necessarily ensure that they achieved a higher standard of knowledge in the biological sciences related to nursing. If the level of knowledge assumed by the doctors in this study is used as a guide, the question arises as to whether, under more favourable conditions, all the nurses in this sample could have reached this standard.

In the present study, the measures used to estimate the general abilities of the nurses were their I.Q. scores and their attainment in school subjects.

In the introduction, the educational level appropriate to entrants to nursing was discussed and it was seen that some nurses, including nurse teachers, have indicated that they consider that the present statutory level should be raised. In the present study it was found that there were wide variations in the correlations between attainment in school subjects and scores in the Science Test. The correlations between the number of passes at higher level and scores of nurses with passes at this level were consistently positive, but there was a substantial relationship between these factors in only one group of nurses.

It could be argued that, if educational attainment considered in isolation is an important factor in the learning of the biological sciences, it would have been demonstrated when the students were working in unfavourable conditions. If conditions were improved, all the students might be expected to achieve a higher standard of knowledge, but the proportion who could reach the level expected of them by doctors is at present a matter for conjecture.

It would seem that further studies are required before reliable information is available regarding the relationship between general educational attainment and different aspects of the theory upon which nursing depends.

Although there was a wide range of intelligence within the total sample of nurses, it was found that I.Q. scores correlated with the scores in the Science Test at the level of +.40 for students and +.55 for staff nurses.

It may be that intelligence testing would be a more reliable guide in the selection of entrants to nursing, so far as their ability in biological sciences is concerned, than attainment in school subjects. There appears to be little encouragement for girls and boys who wish to enter nursing to stay at school until they have attained the maximum number of passes at higher and ordinary level of which they are capable. It would seem that teachers do not encourage pupils who express an interest in nursing to stay at school after they have reached the statutory minimum required for entry to schools of nursing. On this account there may be students entering nursing who would be capable of gaining more passes in school subjects if they stayed longer at school, or if the educational entry standards to nursing were set at a higher level.

There appears to be a need for experiment in nursing education, to study and assess the way in which students perform in a learning environment more favourable than the one which exists at present. It is not known whether students with levels of I.Q. and school attainment similar to those of the nurses in the present study are capable of achieving a higher standard of knowledge in the biological sciences related to nursing. The only British experiment which set out to provide a planned learning environment at basic level, and to assess the students' performance after a shortened period of training, used a sample of students with above-average levels of I.Q. and school attainment (Scott Wright, 1961).

The wide range of ability found among nurses presents obvious teaching problems. It might be possible to group students on admission to the school of nursing according to their levels of intelligence and attainment in school subjects, so that those with approximately the same abilities, so far as abilities can be measured by these methods, would be working in the same group.

The subject content of the programme could be presented at a pace and at a level appropriate to each group, using the methods most likely to stimulate the students' interests. At the end of the course, all students would take the same national examination leading to registration by the General Nursing Council, but it would be hoped that the less able students would have acquired a higher standard than they do under present conditions and that the more able students, and those with the initial advantage of having had a higher level of general education, would have reached a standard well above the required minimum.

However, all nursing knowledge is not of the same kind. There are three major components in a basic nursing programme: (i) that part of nursing which is dependent on the biological sciences; (ii) that part which is dependent on the social sciences; (iii) nursing practice, which is the application of the knowledge derived from both the biological and the social sciences.

Not all students have the same ability and interest in all these areas. If their standard of work appears to be unequal, after they have had time to work in selected groups as suggested above, they could be moved into different classes for different subjects. For example, a student who had no difficulty in understanding the biological science material may have difficulties with the social sciences, or require longer periods of tuition and experience before achieving a satisfactory standard of nursing practice. If students were moved into groups according to their needs, they could work at a pace appropriate to their abilities.

In the introduction it was suggested that it is unlikely that there is a 'standard' type of nurse who can function effectively in any nursing situation. The arrangements suggested above would stimulate the interest of students with the special abilities required to work in certain clinical areas. It is possible that an aptitude for a particular type of scientific study may be linked with an interest in a particular type of nursing. For example, it might be found that nurses who had an aptitude for understanding the biological sciences preferred to work in surgical wards or in intensive care units, while those who showed more ability in social sciences were attacted to community or psychiatric nursing. Such a combination of interests could provide a useful stimulus to teaching and learning, especially in relating theory to practice.

A minimum level of achievement in all three components of the basic nursing programme would be required of all nurses before they were granted registration by the General Nursing Council.

At the present time, students are not permitted to take the final examinations of the General Nursing Council for Scotland until they have completed a total of 144 weeks of nursing study and practice. In the type of situation which has been described, some students may be ready to sit the examination at an earlier date. If this were permitted by the Council, nursing schools could provide opportunities for students to assess their own competence in the theoretical and practical aspects of nursing before deciding whether they wished to present themselves for the final examination. This would also enable the staff of schools of nursing to advise students regarding any areas of study which required special attention. The involvement of the students in making this decision, and the possibility of a reduction in the length of training for students who learned more quickly, could act as an incentive to learning. This arrangement would particularly affect brighter students who are present may become bored with the slow pace at which material is presented.

6.2.4 Teachers of student nurses

If it was decided to raise the standard of nursing education in the biological sciences related to nursing, some consideration would have to be given to the knowledge and ability of the nurses who teach students in the nursing school and in the wards.

In the present study it was found that there was a wide range of ability and knowledge of the biological sciences in the sample of nurses, as demonstrated by I.Q. scores, general educational attainment and scores in the Science Test. It is possible that a similar range of ability exists among the registered nurses who are involved in teaching students.

There would seem to be three main attributes to be considered in relation to teachers, in nursing or in any other subject: firstly, an interest in and commitment to teaching; secondly, the ability to pass on to others the information and attitudes appropriate to the subject matter; thirdly, a sufficient knowledge of the subject matter to be able to select the material appropriate to the students and to the objectives of the course.

Since registered nurse teachers and clinical instructors have elected to specialise in nursing education, it may be assumed that they have an interest in teaching. Both groups have received instruction in how to teach, although clinical instructors have usually studied educational theory and practice at a more superficial level than have registered nurse teachers. As regards their knowledge of the sciences related to nursing, the knowledge of the two groups is likely to vary, depending on their individual abilities and the facilities available for study. Registered nurse teachers, if they have taken a two year preparation for teaching, have had the opportunity to study subject content, including the sciences, to a standard beyond that of the basic nursing syllabus. Clinical instructors, who have a six month course, and those registered nurse teachers who have taken a one year course in a college of education, have had very little opportunity to study the theory related to the material which they teach. Their level of scientific knowledge is therefore likely to be limited unless they have taken further steps to extend it by private study.

The two other groups involved in teaching student nurses are ward sisters and staff nurses. It may generally be assumed that they are willing to accept the responsibility for teaching if they accept appointments to wards to which students are assigned. However, their primary responsibility is to organise and provide patient care and there is little doubt that, by comparison, teaching students has low priority.

The reluctance of ward sisters and staff nurses to teach may be partly due to the fact that they have had no preparation in how to teach. They may also have doubts about the adequacy of their knowledge of the subject matter involved.

There is no doubt that the majority of ward sisters are expert in running their wards and in providing patient care, but they have limited opportunities to raise the level of their theoretical knowledge beyond those provided in their basic nursing training. Some ward sisters and staff nurses have attended post-basic clinical specialist courses, but the majority are dependent upon knowledge acquired from their own reading and observation, and from the doctors with whom they work.

6.2.5 Teaching preparation in basic nurse training

Interest in teaching is obviously desirable in a profession which is concerned with health education and, in order to ensure that all registered nurses have some knowledge of how to teach, it is suggested that elementary instruction, with special emphasis on the methods appropriate to clinical teaching, should be included in the basic nursing programme. This might be done by giving senior students the experience of demonstrating and explaining nursing procedures to junior students, within the setting of the nursing school. In the process of doing so they would develop their teaching abilities and possibly acquire a better understanding of the subjects being taught.

Subsequent teaching preparation would depend to some extent on the professional position of the nurse teacher. The basic training in how to teach should be further developed as part of the preparation of nurses for ward sisters' posts. First line management courses, which at the moment concentrate on the organisation of nursing services at ward level, should be extended to include preparation in how to organise the teaching component of the ward sisters' work.

Of the three factors involved—interest in teaching, teaching ability and knowledge of subject matter—the last named appears to present the greatest problem for staff nurses and ward sisters. In the present study, a variable level of knowledge of the biological sciences was found among staff nurses, and similar variability could be expected among ward sisters.

It would seem that there is a need to provide well organised continuing education programmes which staff nurses and ward sisters would attend during working hours. The objectives of such courses should clearly state that their purpose was to raise the standard of knowledge of the theory upon which nursing depends. If such courses were to be effective, the active participation of those who attended would be essential. Such courses should be financed by Hospital Boards of Management and organised in conjunction with the staff of the school of nursing. It might be necessary to appoint a registered nurse teacher to the nursing service administration staff to organise and coordinate such courses.

It is to be hoped that the long-term effects of continuing education courses of this type would be to improve the standard of patient care.

In the introduction, the concern of a number of writers about the teaching of students by ward sisters and staff nurses was discussed. Environmental factors which prevent these nurses from providing clinical instruction were enumerated, but the ward sisters' interest in teaching was rarely mentioned by these writers as a factor of any importance. The idea that clinical instruction is the 'right' thing to do has been built up over a long period of time, and the ward sister or staff nurse who is frankly not interested in teaching would require to have a great deal of courage to say so.

It would appear that to improve the situation as far as clinical instruction is concerned, a useful first step would be to accept that not all registered nurses are interested in teaching students. It might then be possible to devise a system whereby only those who are interested in teaching would be appointed to wards to which students are assigned.

It would seem that steps need to be taken to establish criteria for the evaluation of clinical instruction. In order to do this studies are needed which could provide information upon which to base these criteria.

At the present time the clinical areas to which student nurses are assigned are approved by the General Nursing Council, but the teaching interest and ability of the ward sisters are not included in the criteria for approval. In fact, when a ward has been approved as suitable for student practice, the ward sister may be changed without reference to the General Nursing Council.

As the Council registers nurse teachers and clinical instructors, it would seem reasonable to suggest that the other registered nurses involved in ward teaching, that is, ward sisters and staff nurses, should have some recognition of their teaching function. If they satisfied the criteria for the teaching of students they could have their registration certificate suitably endorsed and there could be an appropriate salary differential.

6.3 METHODS: SUGGESTED APPLICATION

The methods which were developed for this study could be refined and used in a variety of nursing studies. With appropriate modifications they could be applied to any area of the knowledge upon which nursing depends and to any area of clinical practice.

They could also be used to study the progress of classes of students. Instead of grouping students into 'years' as was done in this study, each intake (at least two a year in the majority of nursing schools) could be considered separately. This would provide the teaching staff with a continuing source of information which would enable them to relate their theoretical teaching to the activities which the students were carrying out in the wards at different stages of their programme. In this way theory and practice could be more closely related, even in the present situation where nurse teachers have virtually no control over the activities assigned to students.

With the kind of information obtained from direct observation in the wards by nurse teachers, the curriculum could be kept up-to-date, not only in relation to the present work of students but also in order to anticipate the changing functions of registered nurses.

The schools of nursing could develop a library of the type of questions used in this study, incorporating the whole range of theoretical knowledge upon which nursing depends. Provided there was a large number of questions, these could be used in different groupings on numerous occasions. Changes would need to be made only to remove questions about activities which the nurses no longer carried out and to add questions which referred to new activities and areas of responsibility.

It is more difficult for the General Nursing Council to keep its syllabus and examination content up-to-date than it is for the schools of nursing to revise their curriculum. Nursing schools could be asked to provide the General Nursing Council with information about changes in nursing practice and about the frequency with which new practices were carried out. Clearly, a 'new' activity which was occasionally carried out in a specialist ward would not necessitate a change in either the syllabus or the examinations, but an accumulation of information from a number of schools might show that a change in the syllabus was justified. This system would provide early indications of the transfer of activities from doctors to nurses.

There was some discussion in the introduction about the definition of the nurses' role. In this study, doctors were included because they are the largest professional group with whom nurses work closely. Similar studies could reveal how physiotherapists, social workers, occupational therapists see the nurses' role, could perhaps assist these paramedical groups to identify their own roles more clearly, and so contribute to the inter-professional understanding and cooperation which is essential to the team concept of patient care.

In the present study the term 'nursing activity' has been used in relation to observable nursing treatments. In a broader sense, it could mean the processes which are involved in decision-making. From the description of the uses which nurses make of information (3.4) it would seem that their managerial functions should receive more careful consideration.

At the present time the study of management as such is not included in the syllabuses of the General Nursing Council for Scotland. It is possible that research could be carried out, applying the methods used in this study, to assist in identifying the management studies which should be included in basic nursing education programmes.

Whatever the methods used to investigate nursing problems, it would seem that a more analytical, less intuitive approach is needed than has been used in the past, particularly in the development of curricula appropriate to the nurse's changing role. A sound background of scientific knowledge would seem to be one of the essential requirements for the registered nurse of the future.

Appendix 1

Nurses' Science Test.

Name

School certificate awarded   Date

Subjects Passed	Higher Grade	Advanced Level	Ordinary Grade/ Level	Lower Grade

---

Question 1

Column A consists of a number of observations which may be made by the nurse assisting the patient to get out of bed. Some of the items in Column B may be causes of the observed abnormalities listed in Column A. Write each number from Column A in the appropriate space in Column B.

No.	Column A	Column B	Place correct no. here
1.	Increase in rate of otherwise normal pulse	Hypertension	
		Atrial fibrillation	
2.	Pallor and dizziness in a patient receiving treatment with hypotensive drugs	Unusual exercise	
		Postural hypotension	
3.	Pale, sweating, rapid weak pulse in post-operation patient	Primary haemorrhage	
		Reactionary haemorrhage	
4.	Acute respiratory distress	Cerebral embolism	
		Heart block	
		Pulmonary embolism	

Question 2

Surgical dressings are commonly performed by nurses. Column A consists of a number of important points of aseptic technique and some of the items in Column B the reasons for their use. Place the number of the item in Column A beside the appropriate reason in Column B.

No. Column A	Column B	Place correct no. here
1. The nurse doing the dressing washes and dries her hands carefully	To prevent contamination of the atmosphere	
2. The soiled dressing is removed with forceps used for that purpose only	Prevents atmospheric contamination of the depths of the wound	
3. Drainage from a wound should be into a closed receptacle.	The organisms may be antibiotic resistant	
4. When a stitch is being removed it should be cut very close to the skin surface	Micro-organisms spread quickly in a moist medium	
5. A dry dressing is preferred to a lotion dressing	Prevents the spread of micro-organisms to the new dressing	
6. Sterile instruments should be used to handle dressings	To develop manual dexterity	
	Antiseptics inhibit the growth of organisms	
	To avoid introducing bacteria from the skin into the deeper layers of tissue	
	Disinfectants kill organisms but damage healthy tissue	
	When many dressings are being done the skin of the hands may become cracked	
	A wound can seal itself from possible infection only when it is dry	
	Instruments can be sterilised but hands can be regarded as sterile only when sterile gloves are worn	

Question 3

The testing of urine for the presence of abnormal constituents is frequently carried out by nurses. Column A consists of some abnormal constituents and Column B some reasons for these abnormalities. Place the number of each item in Column A beside the appropriate reason in Column B..

No.	Column A	Column B	Place correct no. here
1.	Presence of glucose	Reduced permeability of renal capsule	
2.	Presence of acetone	Increased concentration due to increased proportion of dissolved substances	
3.	Specific gravity of 1040 or more		
4.	Presence of albumen	Presence of renal calculi	
5.	Presence of pus	A pyogenic infection of the urinary tract	
		An increase in the permeability of the renal capsule	
		Presence of vaginitis	
		Lack of adrenocorticotropic hormone	
		An increase in the production of the substance	
		Increased intake of the substance	
		Blood level of the substance having risen above the renal threshold	
		Substance not being properly utilised within the body	
		Reduced concentration due to increased water	

Question 4

In preparing a patient for operation under general anaesthesia certain techniques are employed. Column A is a list of some of these techniques, and Column B contains the reasons for their use. Place the number of the item in Column A beside the appropriate reason in Column B.

No. Column A	Column B	Place correct no. here
1. Patient is given nothing to eat or drink before anaesthetic	Indications of kidney damage influence the anaesthetist's choice of anaesthetic	
2. A specimen of urine is tested for the presence of albumen	Patient commonly receives intravenous fluids during anaesthetic, so does not require fluids or nutrition by mouth	
3. Area of operation should be shaved and treated with antiseptic of the surgeon's choice	Prevents possible inhalation of vomitus which may cause pneumonia	
4. Atropine is commonly given three-quarters to one hour before operation	To ensure that the patient's bladder is empty	
5. A narcotic drug is given by injection three-quarters to one hour before operation	To indicate if glucose and insulin should be given before and possibly during operation	
6. A specimen of urine is tested for the presence of sugar and acetone	To indicate the area of operation	
	To reduce the excitability of the patient and facilitate the induction of anaesthesia	
	To inhibit parasympathetic stimulation of the secretary glands of the respiratory and alimentary tracts	
	Slows the rate of contraction of the heart	
	Depresses the respiratory centre	
	To reduce the dangers of wound infection	
	To facilitate respiration during the anaesthetic	

Question 5

Cleaning of the patient's mouth is a nursing practice commonly performed for patients and is usually necessitated by inadequate salivation. Column A consists of some conditions which precipitate the need for mouth care and some of the items in Column B are the underlying reasons. Place the number of each item in Column A beside the appropriate reason in Column B.

No. Column A	Column B	Place correct no. here
1. Patients receiving nourishment by the intravenous route only	Restrictions placed on the position adopted by the patient due to his condition	
2. After severe haemorrhage		
3. In febrile conditions	Tubular reabsorption is inadequate	
4. Acute and chronic diarrhoea	High level of glycosuria	
5. Where there is dysphagia	Generalised dehydration	
6. Patients who sleep with the mouth open	Excessive sweating	
	Fluid does not require to be absorbed	
	Excessive diuresis	
	Loss of electrolytes	
	Excessive thirst	
	Inadequate absorption of water	
	Increased cellular metabolism	
	Difficulty in taking enough food and fluid by mouth	
	Typhoid and paratyphoid fevers	
	Accumulation of urea within the body	
	Expired air is saturated with water vapour	
	The rate of drying exceeds that of salivation	
	Lack of mechanical stimulation	

Question 6

Bathing the patient in the bathroom may expose the patient to the dangers of cross infection. Select from the following list those items which may contribute to cross infection and place a tick beside them in the column provided.

	Place tick here

1. A moist environment is essential for bacterial growth
2. Debris left in the bath by a patient may contain bacteria and nutritional materials which they require for growth
3. The length of time the patient spends in the bath
4. The number of times the patient has bathed in the bathroom
5. The number of patients who use the same bath
6. Patients with wound infections are commonly encouraged to bath as an aid to healing
7. The fact that a dressing requires to be done as soon as the patient has had a bath
8. The disinfectant applied to the bath between patients may have contact with the organisms for only a very short time
9. Towels and toilet requisites left in the bathroom by one patient may provide a source of micro-organisms for others
10. The effectiveness of disinfectants is diminished by the presence of organic material
11. The temperature of the bath water is suitable for the growth of bacteria
12. Patients who have infected wounds are placed at the end of the bathing list

Question 7

Abdominal paracentesis is a treatment performed by the doctor for which the nurse may be asked to prepare the equipment and the patient and assist with the procedure. Column A consists of some points of procedure and Column B the reasons for their use. Place the number of the items in Column A beside the appropriate reason in Column B.

No.	Column A	Column B	Place no. here
1.	The patient's bladder must be known to be empty before treatment begins	Bacteria introduced through the drainage tube may lead to general peritonitis	
2.	The patient should be lying on his back but may require to be supported in a semi-recumbent position	To ensure that the abdominal swelling is not due to a distended bladder	
		To enable the patient to cooperate with the doctor	
3.	Closed drainage should be used	To ensure that all vegetative organisms are killed	
4.	Fluid should be allowed to drain off slowly	Increased intra-abdominal pressure may cause respiratory embarrassment	
5.	All equipment used should be sterilised by steam under pressure	Sudden reduction of pressure on abdominal blood vessels may precipitate severe shock	
		To facilitate siphonage	
		Sporing anaerobic organisms would grow and multiply rapidly in the peritoneal cavity	
		Packs containing all the requirements for this procedure are autoclaved	
		The bladder rises into the abdomen when distended	

Question 8

When a specimen is required for bacteriological examination certain points should receive special attention. Column A consists of a selection of these points, and Column B the reasons for their scientific importance. Place the number of the items in Column A beside the appropriate reason in Column B.

No.	Column A	Column B	Place correct no. here
1.	The specimen is collected in a sterile standard container	So that it will be recognised as a specimen for bacteriological examination	
2.	Chemical substances should not be used to sterilise containers or cleanse the area	The growth and multiplication of organisms will be inhibited but successful culture should be possible	
3.	To provide a specimen of sputum the patient should be instructed to cough into a container whenever he wakes in the morning	Sterilisation by hot air may damage the container	
4.	Specimens not being sent to the laboratory immediately should be kept in a cool place	To facilitate antibiotic and sulphonamide sensitivity tests	
		Accumulated secretions are likely to contain infecting organisms	
5.	The specimen should not come in direct contact with the hands of the nurse	Patient is rested and therefore finds it easier to provide a specimen	
6.	Specimens should be collected before chemotherapeutic drugs are administered	To avoid cross infection	
		To prevent contamination of the specimen	
		May prevent the growth of organisms on culture media	
		To prevent growth of the organisms before culture	
		May make culture of organisms difficult	

Question 9

Prevention of the development of pressure sores is an important part of nursing care. Column A consists of some of the methods of doing so, and Column B the reasons for their success. Place the number of the items in Column A in the appropriate place in Column B.

No.	Column A	Column B	Place correct no. here
1.	Frequent change of the position of the patient	To distribute the pressure over a wider area away from the bony prominences	
2.	Changing linen, washing and drying of the area contaminated if the patient is incontinent	To relieve pressure on sensory nerve endings	
3.	Early ambulation	To allow the skin time to heal	
4.	Special attention to the diet, especially protein and vitamin content	General improvement of cell nutrition	
		Improves general circulation	
5.	Use of air rings, woolrings, slings and pulleys if patient must remain in one position	In preparation for the application of ointment	
		Helps to prevent chest and urinary complications	
		Improves appetite	
		Decomposing urine produces ammonia which predisposes to infection	
		To make the patient more comfortable	
		Improvement of the blood circulation in arterioles and capiliaries in the pressure area	

Question 10

In Column A there is a list of conditions necessary for the sterilisation of equipment by steam under pressure (autoclaving). In Column B there are the reasons for successful sterilisation by this method. Write the number of the item in Column A beside the appropriate reason in Column B.

No.	Column A	Column B	Place correct no. here
1.	Steam is used	Moist heat sterilises more efficiently	
2.	Pressure greater than atmospheric pressure is used	Different rates of expansion of the parts may lead to breakages	
3.	Wrapping materials permeable to steam are used	Sterilisation begins when the desired temperature is reached at the centre of the packet	
4.	Facilities are provided for drying sterilised materials in the autoclave	Forces the steam to the centre of the packet	
5.	Syringes are packed with the barrel and plunger separated	Only surfaces in contact with steam are sterilised	
6.	The time of exposure is supervised	The temperature increases with the pressure	
		Steam does not damage the materials to be sterilised	
		Bacteria do not penetrate dry materials easily	
		It is more convenient to use dry sterile materials	
		Steam can penetrate to the middle of a packet	
		Steam sterilises at a lower temperature than air	
		Plastic materials used for wrapping prevent contamination after sterilisation	

Question 11

Patients in hospital are weighed for a variety of reasons. Place a tick beside the valid reasons in the following list

	Place tick here
1. To calculate the body surface area for the estimation of the basal metabolic rate	
2. To indicate the effect of treatment of gastro-intestinal disorders	
3. To indicate progress in the treatment of rheumatic heart disease	
4. To indicate progress in the treatment of pernicious anaemia	
5. To indicate the cardiac output	
6. To calculate the dose of histamine for a histamine secretion test	
7. To indicate the effect of treatment for severe shock	
8. To indicate the effect of treatment with thiouracil	
9. Before and after treatment with diuretic drugs	
10. As an accurate measure of changes in the amount of oedema	

Question 12

The taking of blood pressure at regular intervals is a procedure commonly prescribed for patients in hospital. Place a tick beside those physiological factors in the following list which influence the blood pressure level.

	Place tick here
1. The electrolyte balance in the body	
2. The effectiveness of the venous return to the heart	
3. The degree of bronchial constriction	
4. The viscosity of the blood	
5. The state of constriction of the small arteries and arterioles	
6. The acid-base balance of the body	
7. The urinary output	
8. The rate of contraction of the heart	
9. The volume of blood ejected from the heart with each contraction of the ventricles	
10. The amount of fluid intake and output	
11. The effectiveness of lymphatic drainage	
12. The body temperature	
13. The volume of blood in circulation	

Question 13

Bladder irrigation and drainage is commonly employed in the post operation care of patients who had had the prostate gland removed. Column A consists of some of the factors to be considered in arranging the supervising this treatment and Column B contains the reasons for these factors. Place the number of each item in Column A beside the appropriate reason in Column B.

No.	Column A	Column B	Place correct no. here
1.	The height of the bottle of irrigating fluid	Results in leakage round the abdominal tube	
2.	The rate of flow of the irrigating fluid	Indicates the amount of urine secreted	
3.	An increase in the flow of fluid without a corresponding increase in drainage	To facilitate siphonage	
		Relieves the tension within the bladder	
4.	The tube leading from the bladder should be above the level of the fluid in the receptacle	May indicate blockage of the siphoning tube by blood clot	
		Indicates blockage of the tube leading into the bladder	
5.	Irrigating bottle should not be allowed to run empty	Indicates the amount of fluid entering the bladder	
6.	The fluid entering the bladder and withdrawn from it should be measured	Indicates the pressure of fluid entering the bladder	
		Indicates distension of the bladder	
		Indicates the rate of siphonage	
		Siphonage requires that the tube from the bladder is full of fluid	
		Shows the capacity of the bladder	

Question 14

Sterilisation by boiling. A recognised technique of sterilisation by boiling is carried out in hospital wards. In Column A there is a list of some of the steps of this technique, and in Column B a list of possible reasons for taking these steps. Place the number of each step from Column A beside the appropriate reason in Column B.

No.	Column A	Column B	Place correct no. here
1.	Rinse in cold water	Low temperature prevents the growth of organisms	
2.	Wash in warm soapy water		
3.	Boil in 2% sodium carbonate solution in preference to tap water	Ensures articles remain sterile	
		To prevent the nurse burning herself	
4.	Completely immerse articles to be sterilised	Grease leaves a scum on the sides of the steriliser	
5.	Boiling for three to five minutes is adequate	The temperature of the boiling liquid is constant while that of the mixture of the air and steam above the surface is variable	
6.	Sterile forceps are used to remove articles from the steriliser	To act as an antiseptic and inhibit the growth of organisms	
		To remove organic material without causing coagulation	
		Kills all organisms	
		Acts as a detergent	
		Boiling temperature higher than 100°C	
		Kills vegitative organisms	
		The temperature of steam and water at atmospheric pressure are the same	

Question 15

Treatment of the eyes by irrigation, administration of drugs in the form of eye drops and ointments is frequently carried out in general hospital wards. Column A consists of some points of technique and Column B some reasons why these points are important. Place the number from Column A beside the appropriate reason in Column B.

No.	Column A	Column B	Place correct no. here
1.	Eyelids and eyelashes should be gently swabbed before irrigation commences	The temperature of an exposed surface is lower than that in the mouth	
2.	The head should be tilted backwards and to the affected side	To give the patient confidence	
		To prevent contamination of the remaining material	
3.	Temperature of irrigating fluid should be about 95°F	So that the total amount of drug can be introduced at one time	
4.	Drops should be instilled into the lower conjunctival sac	To eliminate any danger of burning the patient	
5.	When ointment is being administered all the ointment to be used should be taken on the applicator at one time	The drug will be absorbed before being squeezed out of the eye	
		Less painful for the patient	
		To remove organisms and grit which may be introduced with the irrigating fluid	
		To prevent washing infected material into the other eye	
		The receiver for the fluid is held at the side of the head	

Question 16

The prescription of intravenous fluids for a patient is 3 bottles of 0.9% sodium chloride and 3 bottles of 5% glucose in 24 hours. Each bottle contains 500 ml. How many drops per minute will be necessary to ensure that the 3 litres of fluid extend over the required period of time?

Underline the correct answer

17
21
25
30
35
39
43
47
53
57
61

Question 17

A specific blood concentration of a drug must be maintained in order to provide effective treatment of the condition from which the patient is suffering. Place a tick beside those factors in the following list which affect the blood concentration of the drug.

	Place tick here
1. The rate of absorption from the alimentary tract	
2. The toxicity of the drug	
3. The size of the patient	
4. The volume of urine excreted	
5. The amount of exercise taken by the patient	
6. The frequency of dosage	
7. The fact that the drug acts selectively on some tissues and not on others	
8. The solubility of the drug in the body fluids.	
9. The rate of excretion of the drug	
10. The ability of the liver to destroy the drug	

Question 18

If a patient has had a haemorrhage the pulse rate will be markedly increased. Select from the following list the reasons for this and place a tick beside them in the space provided.

	Place tick here
1. To compensate for the reduction in volume of the circulating blood	
2. To encourage an increase in blood volume by the passage of tissue fluid into the blood vessels	
3. To increase the output of urine and the excretion of urea	
4. Because the venous return is reduced	
5. To facilitate the excretion of carbon dioxide	
6. Because the output of the heart with each beat is reduced	
7. To meet the demands of the muscles for an increase in the supply of oxygen and nutrient materials	
8. Because of the reflex effect of reduced blood pressure	
9. Because the reduced blood volume will flow more easily through the blood vessels	
10. In order to keep pace with the increased respiration rate	
11. There will be less resistance to the flow of blood because of the reduced viscosity	
12. The amount of haemoglobin available to transport oxygen will be reduced	

Question 19

Column A consists of a list of drugs which have been provided by the pharmaceutical department, with the labels indicating strength in imperial measure. Column B consists of a variety of metric measures. Place the number of each item in Column A beside the equivalent metric measure in Column B.

No.	Column A	Column B	Place correct no. here
1.	Ephedrine, ½ grain tablet	0.02 mg	
2.	Omnopon, 1/3 grain ampoule	0,05 mg	
3.	Atropine, 1/100 grain ampoule	0.20 mg	
4.	Sodium Amytal, 1½ grain capsules	0.40 mg	
5.	Hyoscine, 1/150 grain ampoule	0.60 mg	
6.	Morphine, ¼ grain ampoule	0.80 mg	
		1.00 mg	
		5.00 mg	
		10.00 mg	
		15.00 mg	
		20.00 mg	
		25.00 mg	
		30.00 mg	
		35.00 mg	
		45.00 mg	
		75.00 mg	
		80.00 mg	
		90.00 mg	
		110.00 mg	
		120.00 mg	

Appendix II

Doctors' Questionnaire and Correspondence

Please tick the position you hold in the National Health Service and state the length of time you have been employed at this level.

	House Officer	Registrar	Consultant

If there are any comments which you would like to make about the questionnaire please write them on this sheet.

Question 1

The following is a list of some observations and possible reasons for them which might be made by the staff nurse when assisting a patient to get out of bed. Do you consider that she should have this knowledge to assist her in deciding the urgency of her report to the medical staff?

Yes   No

1. An increase in the rate of an otherwise normal pulse may be due to unusual exercise
2. Pallor and dizziness may be due to postural hypotension in a patient receiving drug treatment for hypertension
3. Pallor, sweating, rapid weak pulse in the post operation period may be due to reactionary haemorrhage
4. Acute respiratory distress may be due to pulmonary embolism

Question 2

Surgical dressings are treatments commonly performed or supervised by the staff nurse. Place a tick beside those items with which you consider the staff nurse should be familiar, without specific prescription, if she is responsible for this work.

Place tick here

1. The nurse doing the dressing washes and dries her hands to prevent the easy spread of organisms in a moist medium

2. That soiled dressings are removed with forceps used for that purpose only in order to prevent the contamination of the new dressing

3. That drainage of a wound should be into a closed receptacle to prevent contamination of the depths of the wound

4. When a stitch is being removed it is cut very close to the skin to prevent the introduction of bacteria from the skin into the deeper layers of tissue

5. That a dry dressing and access to the air is preferred to a moist closed dressing to encourage the wound to seal itself

6. That sterile instruments should be used to handle dressing and not the hands as the hands can never be considered as sterile unless sterile gloves are worn

Question 3

Testing urine is a technique frequently performed or supervised by the staff nurse. The following is a list of abnormalities which may be found, with some fundamental reasons for them. Place a tick beside those items which you consider would influence the urgency of her report to you (assuming her full knowledge of the management of the patient).

Place tick here

1. That glucose is present because it has exceeded the renal threshold level

2. That acetone is present in untreated or unstable diabetes mellitus because of an increase in its production

3. That 1041 is a high specific gravity due to an increase in the proportion of dissolved substances in the urine

4. That albumen is present because of disease within the kidney which has increased the permeability of the glomerular membrane

5. That pus is present because of pyogenic infection of the urinary tract

Question 4

When a patient is being prepared for operation under general anaesthetic certain points of procedure require special attention. Place a tick beside the items in the following list which you consider the staff nurse should initiate.

Place tick here

1. The patient is given nothing to eat or drink for at least six hours before a general anaesthetic to reduce the danger of inhalation pneumonia

2. The patient's urine is tested for albumen, as evidence of kidney damage might influence the anaesthetist's choice of anaesthetic

3. The area of operation should be treated with the antiseptic of the surgeon's choice to reduce the possibility of wound infection

4. The prescribed pre-operation medication to limit the respiratory and gastric secretions should be given three quarters to one hour before operation

5. The prescribed pre-operation narcotic, to reduce the excitability of the patient and facilitate the induction of anaesthesia, should be given three-quarters to one hour before operation

6. The urine should be tested for sugar and acetone, to indicate if glucose and insulin should be given before and possibly during operation

Question 5

The following is a list of situations in which oral hygiene is an important part of nursing care. Place a tick beside those items in which you consider the staff nurse should initiate oral hygiene without specific prescription.

Place tick here

1. Where there is lack of mechanical stimulation of salivation because the patient is receiving only intravenous fluids and nutrients

2. In general dehydration as a result of severe haemorrhage

3. Where there is excessive sweating due to high temperature

4. Where there is inadequate absorption of water in acute and chronic diarrhoea

5. Where there is dysphagia causing difficulty in taking enough food and fluid by mouth

6. Where sleeping with the mouth open results in the rate of drying of the epithelium exceeding the rate of salivation

Question 6

Bathing patients in the bathroom may be a prescribed treatment for some patients. Place a tick beside the items in the following list which you consider the staff nurse should understand in order to prevent possible cross infection by this route.

Place tick here

1. That the moist atmosphere in the bathroom is consistent with bacterial growth

2. That cell debris which may accumulate in the bath may contain pathogenic micro-organisms and nutritional materials which they require for growth

3. That there is a danger that disinfectant applied to the bath between patients may have contact with the micro-organisms for only a very short time

4. That the effectiveness of disinfectants is diminished by the presence of organic material

5. The temperature of the bath water is suitable for the growth of micro-organisms

Question 7

Preparing the equipment and the patient for abdominal paracentesis is an activity carried out or supervised by the staff nurse. Place a tick beside those items with which you consider the staff nurse should be familiar, without specific prescription if she is responsible for this work.

Place tick here

1. The patient's bladder must be known to be empty because it rises into the abdomen when distended

2. The patient should lie on his back but may require to be supported in a semi-recumbent position, as increased intra-abdominal pressure may cause respiratory embarrassment

3. Closed drainage should be used as micro-organisms introduced through the drainage tube may lead to general peritonitis

4. The peritoneal fluid should drain slowly, as a sudden reduction in the pressure on abdominal blood vessels may precipitate severe shock

5. All the equipment used should be sterilised by steam under pressure as sporing anaerobic organisms would grow and multiply rapidly in the peritoneal cavity

Question 8

The following is a list of precautions which should be taken in the collection of specimens for bacteriological examination. Place a tick beside those which you consider should be applied by the staff nurse without specific prescription.

Place tick here

1. The specimen should be collected in a sterile standard container
2. Chemical substances should not be used to sterilise containers or cleanse the area
3. Specimens of sputum should be *coughed* up
4. Specimens not being sent to the laboratory immediately should be kept in a cool place
5. The specimen should not come in direct contact with the hands of the nurse
6. If a chemotherapeutic drug has been prescribed the specimen should be collected before it is administered

Question 9

Place a tick beside the items of preventive care of pressure areas in the following list which you consider the staff nurse should initiate without specific prescription.

Place tick here

1. Frequent change of position of the patient
2. Changing linen, washing and drying of the area if it is contaminated if the patient is incontinent
3. Early ambulation if there are no contraindications
4. Special attention to the diet especially the protein and vitamin content
5. The use of air rings, wool rings, slings and pulleys if the patient must remain in one position

Question 10

When you ask a staff nurse to prepare equipment for an aseptic technique, e.g. marrow puncture, for which the materials have to be sterilised by steam under pressure, is it your practice to prescribe the following details of method of sterilisation if central supply is not available?

Yes   No

1. The temperature and pressure of the steam
2. The type of wrapping or container used
3. That the materials are dried after sterilisation
4. The syringes are packed with the barrel and plunger separated
5. The time of exposure of the articles to steam

Question 11

Place a tick beside the conditions in the following list in which you would expect the staff nurse to initiate weight recording without specific prescription.

Place tick here

1. Before the estimation of basal metabolism
2. In gastro-intestinal dysfunction
3. Before histamine secretion test
4. When a patient is being treated with thiouracil
5. Before and after treatment with diuretic drugs
6. As an accurate measure of changes in the amount of oedema

Question 12

The following is a list of factors which influence the blood pressure level. Place a tick beside those items with which you consider the staff nurse should be familiar, if she is responsible for taking and recording the blood pressure of patients in your charge.

Place tick here

1. That the cardiac output depends upon the venous return and the efficiency of the heart as a pump
2. That the viscosity of the blood may be altered in severe shock and burns
3. That the state of dilation of the arterioles may be influenced by drugs or surgery in the treatment of hypertension
4. That the volume of circulating blood may be altered by haemorrhage and shock

Question 13

On your return to the ward after an operating session which began with a prostatectomy would you expect to find that the staff nurse had set the patient up on the type of bladder drainage or irrigation and drainage which you prescribed before leaving the ward? Please tick the appropriate answer.

If your answer is 2 please give examples.

1. Always
2. Sometimes
3. Never

Question 14

Some equipment used in the wards is sterilised by boiling. Do you consider that the staff nurse should be responsible for the supervision of this procedure? Please tick the appropriate answer.

If your answer is 2 please give examples.

    1.   Always
    2.   Sometimes
    3.   Never

Question 15

If a patient in a general hospital ward requires to have his eyes treated by irrigation, administration of a drug in the form of drops or ointment, would you prescribe the method *by which this should be done if there is a qualified nurse on duty? Please tick the appropriate answer*

If it is 2 please give examples.

    1.   Always
    2.   Sometimes
    3.   Never

Question 16

A patient in your care is on intravenous fluids and under the supervision of the staff nurse of the ward. Please indicate in the following example, by placing a tick beside it, your customary method *of prescription of alternate bottles of 5% glucose and 0.9% sodium chloride four hourly for a 24 hour period.*

1. Alternate 500 ml bottles of 0.9% sodium chloride and 5% glucose, total—3 bottles of each

2. Alternate bottles of 0.9% sodium chloride and 5% glucose four hourly

3. 500 ml bottles of 0.9% sodium chloride and 5% glucose alternately

4. Other method... please give example

Question 17

A patient is on sulphonamide therapy for the treatment of a condition which necessitates the maintenance of a therapeutic blood level of the drug. The following is a list of circumstances in which the dose could not be administered or retained at the prescribed time. Place a tick beside those occasions in which you consider the staff nurse should initiate the restoration of the therapeutic blood level of the drug. •

Place tick here

1. Because the patient has just vomited a dose
2. The 2 a.m. dose was omitted because the patient was asleep
3. The patient was absent from the ward for some diagnostic or therapeutic reason
4. The patient was being prepared for another test and not allowed to take anything by mouth

Question 18

If the staff nurse found that a post-operation patient with a rapid weak pulse had a falling blood pressure should she prepare for blood transfusion while someone else called you to the ward?

If your answer is 2 please give examples.

1. Always
2. Sometimes
3. Never

Question 19

Some drugs may be prescribed in metric measure and dispensed in imperial measure or vice versa. If such a drug is prescribed would you consider it the responsibility of the staff nurse in charge of the ward to ensure that the patient received the dose?

1. Always
2. Sometimes
3. Never

Nursing Studies Unit,
University of Edinburgh,
19 Chalmers Street,
Edinburgh.

Dear

In the past two years I have been studying the work of student nurses and staff nurses in hospital wards. Part of this time has been spent in (name of hospital) where everyone has been most cooperative.

I am particularly interested in the staff nurse and her preparation. At this stage it would be of considerable value to have the views and opinions of physicians and surgeons on the basic knowledge and understanding which she has of a number of practical situations.

The attached questionnaire, which I hope you will complete and return to me, consists of a sample of activities which are frequently performed by nurses and I would welcome your views on some aspects of these nursing duties.

I should be grateful if you would not discuss the questionnaire with your nursing and medical colleagues as it is your views which I am anxious to have at this stage.

If there are any questions or commentary I shall be glad to discuss it with you.

Yours sincerely,

Kathleen J. W. Wilson
Lecturer

Nursing Studies Unit,
University of Edinburgh,
19 Chalmers Street,
Edinburgh.

Dear

Towards the end of November you received a questionnaire concerned with a research project on the sciences of nursing.

Already there has been a good response from the medical staff of (name of hospital) and, as a wide variety of opinion has been expressed, I am most anxious to have your contribution.

I fully realise that there are great demands on your time but the successful conclusion of this study depends, to a large extent, on your help.

I hope you will be able to complete the questionnaire and return it to me in the near future.

Yours sincerely,

Kathleen J. W. Wilson
Lecturer

Appendix III

Report of the Committee on Nursing

In 1972, after this thesis was completed, the Report of the Committee on Nursing was published. This report has been accepted in principle by the Government but, in order to implement the recommendations, changes will need to be made in the legislation governing nursing education. At the present time there is no information available regarding the timetabling of such legislation or whether all the recommendations will be accepted.

The terms of reference of this Committee were as follows:

To review the role of the nurse and the midwife in the hospital and the community and the education and training required for that role, so that the best use is made of available manpower to meet present needs and the needs of an integrated health service.

The only recommendations of the Committee which will be considered here are those which have a direct or indirect bearing on the subject of this thesis, that is, those which may influence the teaching and learning of the biological sciences:

1. the form of the nursing education programme
2. the educational requirement for entry to nursing and the minimum age of entry to nursing
3. the employee status of student nurses
4. teaching in the clinical situation.

Under each of these headings the relevant passages from the Briggs report are quoted, and then discussed in relation to the findings of the present study.

Form of nursing education programme recommended

The Committee proposed that the present programmes leading to enrolment and to registration should merge during the first 18 months of training.

Once students have been accepted, we believe that there are great advantages both from an educational and from a social point of view in initiating all of them to the profession through the medium of one basic course. This course would contain a common core of clinical experience but there would be scope for limited options. Within the framework of the course students should be able to develop their theoretical knowledge according to their ability. We have tried to outline the shortest possible course which will produce a safe and confident practical nurse. The basic qualifications for all students at the end of such a course, whatever their qualifications at entry, will be a Certificate in Nursing Practice. The objectives of all courses leading up to the acquisition of this Certificate should be:

a. to provide experience and related teaching in the basic nursing skills;
b. to provide experience and related teaching in the nursing of patients with physical,

mental and behavioural disorders, in the nursing of patients of different age groups and levels of dependency and, of equal importance, in the nursing of patients in both hospital and community settings. (Para. 270).

It is recommended that there should be a four-week introductory course and that:

Following this introductory course nursing students would puruse a programme of study and work related to a core of four twelve-week 'modules'... We believe that the 'modular' system enables the individual through the study of units of experience and related teaching gradually to build up knowledge and skills and acquire a deeper and larger understanding of the practice of nursing. (Para. 275).

The four twelve-week modules would comprise experience in each of the four main clinical areas of medical, surgical, psychiatric and community nursing, and in each module theory and practice would be dealt with concurrently; additionally there would be at least twenty weeks' further clinical experience... We feel certain that with this experience behind them Certificated nurses will thereafter be able to perform adequately at the basic level in the nursing team in any field (Para. 276).

All students should have the equivalent of two weeks out of the twelve weeks spent on each module safeguarded exclusively for education. Determining the use and distribution of this time would be a matter for the Colleges of Nursing and Midwifery, but in every case the time set aside should provide for:

   a. an introduction to new areas of clinical experience;
   b. an element of continuing teaching during clinical experience;
   c. an opportunity for the student to summarise knowledge acquired and to clarify subjects not completely understood (Para. 278).

After receiving the Certificate of Nursing Practice some nurses may continue to undertake a further 18 months' preparation.

We recommend that students who have the ability and the desire to train further after completing their statutory Certificate in Nursing Practice would apply to proceed through the next 18 months to Registration. We see great value in also providing during this period a more academically demanding course which would lead to the award of a Higher Certificate as well as Registration. This dual course would be particularly suitable for those nursing students who had shown above-average ability in the course for the Certificate in Nursing Practice (Para. 285).

It is suggested that the part of the course leading to Registration should consist of three modules followed by nursing practice in one or two clinical settings. There is no recommendation regarding either the duration of these modules or the amount of time which should be allocated to the study of the theory upon which nursing depends.

Students may study for a Higher Certificate either during the second 18 months of the Registration programme or at any time thereafter.

We recommend that the courses for the Higher Certificate should last six months. This Certificate would provide an additional qualification for the nurse. An 18 month course leading to the dual qualification might take the form of two Registration course modules followed by the six-month course for the Higher Certificate (which would include the third module) followed by one or two units of clinical experience (Para. 296).

The Committee has emphasised that nursing education should be a continuing process and that provision should be made for easy transfer

from one specialist area of nursing to another by studying further modules at either Registration or Higher Certificate level at any time following their initial Registration.

We wish to stress that Registration is not the end of the story for the modern nurse and midwife or for the nurse and midwife of the future. The education of nurses and midwives is a continuous process... knowledge and the social context are changing and new experience can and must be acquired beyond this stage. This approach to learning is fundamental to our proposals. The objective of education is to raise the quality of patient care. It is the quality of the education which concerns us, not the possession of more and more formal certificates. (Para. 300).

The suggested content of the course leading to Certification appears to provide students with little opportunity to learn the biological sciences, or any other theory upon which nursing depends, as it is recommended that only two weeks in each 12 week module should be 'safe-guarded exclusively for education'. It would seem therefore that students are likely to be asked to carry out nursing activities without having acquired the associated knowledge of biological sciences, unless they have studied these subjects before entering nursing or background theory is very skillfully incorporated into teaching in the clinical situation.

As these students will be regarded as nursing service personnel, trained staff in charge of wards will be dependent upon them to provide the nursing care required by the patients, observe the effects of medical and nursing treatments and report what they consider to be significant observations. It is difficult to see how they can select the observations to be reported without having a knowledge of first, human biology, second, the patients' abnormalities, third, the aims of medical and nursing treatment and fourth the complications which may develop during or following treatment.

From the point of view of the care of the patients it would seem that safeguards will need to be established to ensure that Certificated nurses will be expected to work only at a level which is consistent with their limited theoretical knowledge.

In the modules leading to Registration and the award of Higher Certificates the Committee has made no suggestion about the amount of time which should be allocated to theoretical study. However, it is recommended that:

The different elements in the Higher Certificate course would be studied in greater depth than subjects either in the curriculum of the Certificate in Nursing Practice or in the modules leading to Registration. (Para. 297).

The amount of time to be 'safeguarded exclusively for education' between Certification and Registration, and the level of knowledge expected of nurses who attain Registration, will presumably have to be decided by the statutory body. Nurse tutors will, no doubt, continue to be free to set higher standards if they so wish.

In the foregoing research it was found that the doctors expected staff nurses to have a greater depth of knowledge of the biological sciences than the staff nurses displayed in the Science Test. In the discussion on this finding it was suggested that 'a decision to raise the standard of the staff nurses' knowledge of the biological sciences related to nursing would have implications for the basic programme of nursing education' (section 6.2.1).

It is not known whether similar findings would be obtained if the study were repeated at this time. If similar findings were obtained and it was considered desirable that students' level of knowledge of the biological sciences should be raised, the recommendations for the second 18 months of the Registration programme are sufficiently permissive to allow for the appropriate emphasis to be placed on the theoretical content of the modules.

Educational attainment before entering nursing and age of entry

The Committee does not recommend a minimum standard of educational attainment for entry to nursing. It makes the point that:

... it will be necessary to recruit from applicants with different initial academic qualifications, ranging from average intelligence to the highest... (Para. 259).

The report goes on to recommend that there should be an increase in the university facilities for basic nursing education and that the educational qualifications for entry to these courses should be decided by the university concerned; that there will be a need to attract applicants with 'A' level passes and a larger number with at least 4 'O' level passes or their equivalent.

In relation to educational achievement the Committee makes the point that:

... as is the case with so many other careers, the relationship between secondary school performance and success in nursing and midwifery is still uncertain. While, therefore, we wish to draw attention to the need to attract candidates who have "done well" at school, we believe that nursing often appeals strongly to late developers and to people with average intelligence or more who, though they have few formal academic qualifications, have a high degree of motivation. Suitability should not be determined by O levels alone. (Para. 259e).

The Committee states, in paragraph 270, 'that there are great advantages both from an educational and a social point of view' in having only one portal of entry to nursing. It does not explain what these advantages are but it may be justifiable to assume that they are the same as those which are associated with the comprehensive school system in general education.

As in the comprehensive schools, this will mean that teachers in Colleges of Nursing will have within each group, students with very different academic and intellectual ability, especially in the course leading to the award of the Certificate in Nursing Practice.

However, the major difference between the comprehensive school system and the Committee's proposals is that of *time for the teachers to teach and the students to learn.* The students, in the 78 week course leading to Certification, will have only 12 weeks available exclusively for educational purposes and these will be divided into a minimum of four separate periods of study. With this amount and distribution of time at their disposal nurse teachers may find it difficult to organise and provide learning experiences in ways which are appropriate to the different abilities of the students in each group. Those students at the lower end of the range of ability may find it difficult to keep up with the course and those at the upper end may experience insufficient intellectual stimulation to sustain their interest in nursing.

The alternative route by which students with sufficient passes in the S.C.E. and G.C.E. examinations may enter nursing is through basic nursing education programmes offered by technical colleges in Scotland, by polytechnics in England and Wales and by universities. The Committee's recommendation that these facilities should be increased may result in some 'creaming off' of candidates with high academic attainment from the National Health Service Colleges of Nursing. This would make the teaching in the Colleges of Nursing easier because the students they recruit would be at the lower end and in the middle of the range of ability, plus a smaller number of very able students who left school without taking S.C.E. or G.C.E. examinations.

If the statutory level of education for entry to nursing is very low or unspecified, some students who could obtain passes at Higher level in the S.C.E. or at 'A' level in the G.C.E. may decide that it is unnecessary to do so. Later they may be disappointed to find that they are not eligible for admission to institutions of higher education where tutors, administrators and researchers are prepared.

The Committee proposes that the minimum age of entry to nursing should be lowered to 17 years. This, together with the Committee's statements on the educational requirements for entry to nursing, may influence the career advice given to pupils in secondary school by teachers and careers advisors. It would be understandable if they decide that nursing is a suitable career for their less able pupils and that more able pupils need not stay at school to obtain Higher level passes in the S.C.E. or 'A' level passes in the G.C.E. unless they wish to enter institutions of higher education.

A view of the literature and discussion of the findings in the foregoing study which refer to educational attainment are available in sections 1.4.4, 5.1, 5.2, 5.4 and 6.2.3.

Employment status of students

The Committee on Nursing, like previous commissions, working parties and writers since 1932, (section 1.3.3) took evidence on, and considered the question of, the employee status of student nurses. With the notable exception of such writers as Balme (1937) and Carter (1939), the Committee on Nursing reached the same conclusion as its predecessors in recommending that the employee status of student nurses should remain unchanged.

A number of bodies recommended to us that responsibilities and powers for nurse and midwife education should be transferred from the Health Departments to the Education Departments... we do not favour such a transfer, although we would welcome continued consultation between these Departments. We believe that it is only within the Health Departments, which are concerned with manpower forecasting and manpower deployment, that educational policies can properly be related to long-term manpower needs, and we consider it essential that Departmental projections prepared in the manpower and personnel units should be discussed regularly with the Central Council to ensure a common approach. (Para. 649).

At this time it is not clear how the student nurses' programme will be affected by the nursing service needs of their employers. The Committee recommends that:

As far as possible, nursing students should be allowed to choose the type of experience covered in their first module. Thereafter the modules could be taken in any order according to local circumstances. (Para. 277).

It will be necessary for the nursing service administrators to work closely with the Colleges of Nursing to establish for each clinical area the number and seniority of students who can be taught and supervised by trained staff. The presence of too many students in a clinical area could be detrimental to patient care in that area and to the students' learning. These principles would apply whether students were employees or not but the recommendation is sufficiently permissive to allow for a wide variety of interpretations. The modules could be arranged to meet the nursing service needs rather than the educational needs of the students.

A review of the literature and discussion of the findings in the foregoing study which refer to the subject of the employee status of student nurses are available in sections 1.3.3 and 6.2. As no change has been recommended the arguments presented in section 6.2 would seem to continue to be relevant.

Teaching in the clinical situation

In the type of programme outlined above a large part of the teaching of student nurses will take place in the clinical situation. It was suggested earlier that very skilful teaching will be required if background theory is to be incorporated into clinical teaching.

The shortage of trained tutors was recognised by the Committee in its recommendation that there is an urgent need to increase their numbers. However, as little progress has been made in this direction so far, it would seem that the main burden of teaching in the clinical situation will remain with the nursing service staff. This subject was discussed in section 6.2 of the foregoing thesis where concern was expressed regarding the facilities which are available for nursing service staff to advance their knowledge of the theory upon which nursing depends and to acquire teaching expertise.

One of the findings of a personal survey carried out for the Committee would seem to justify this concern. A sample of 3027 trainees and recently trained nurses were asked to name which aspect of training in their view most needed improving' and the aspect mentioned by the highest proportion of respondents (32 per cent) was 'the quality of teaching on the wards'. (Para. 219).

No recommendation has been made by the Committee which is likely to improve the quality of teaching by nursing service staff in the short term.

At the present time a good deal of thought is being given to the organisational feasibility of the Briggs Committee's recommendations, and the implications for nursing service. An equal amount of thought will be required to determine their *educational* feasibility, and their long-term effects upon the standard of nursing care.

REFERENCES

Anderson, J.A.D. & Draper, P.A. (1967) The attachment of local authority staff to general practices. *The Medical Officer,* **117**, 111-114.

Arthure, H.G.E. (1970) Responsibilities of doctors and midwives. (Correspondence) *British Medical Journal,* ii, 790.

Balme, H. (1937) *A criticism of nursing education,* p. 17. London: Oxford University Press.

Beck, F. (1958) *Basic nursing education* pp. 42-43. London: International Council of Nurses.

Bird, H.C.H. (1968) Nursing service in general practice. (Correspondence) *British Medical Journal,* i, 378-379.

Boddy, F.A. (1969) *The General Practitioner's View of the Home Nursing Service,* (a) p.2 (b) pp.2, 13 (c) p.22. Department of Public Health and Social Medicine. University of Aberdeen. Unpublished.

Bowers, D.M. (1970) Why not teach nursing to doctors? *Nursing Times,* **66**, No. 1, 24.

British Medical Journal (1967) Nurses and doctors. *British Medical Journal Supplement* 8.4.67, 15-16.

British Medical Journal (1967) Resuscitation and the nurse. (Leading article) ii, 65.

British Medical Journal (1970) Seebohm sequel. (Leading article) iv, 254-255.

British Medical Journal (1970) Unheard voices: the paediatrician, ii, 171-172.

Burkett, R. (1970) Staffing of casualty departments. (Correspondence) *British Medical Journal,* iii, 585.

Carstairs, V. (1966) *Home nursing in Scotland.* Scottish Health Service Studies No. 2. Edinburgh: Scottish Home and Health Department.

Carter, G.B. (1939) *A New Deal for Nurses,* p. 149. London: Gollancz.

Catnach, A. & Houghton, M. (1961) *Report on pilot investigation into methods of teaching in nurse-training schools,* p.19. London: South-West Metropolitan Area Nurse Training Committee.

Conran. M. (1970) Hospital nursing—problems and solutions. *Guy's Hospital Gazette,* **84**, 483-490.

Crichton, A. & Crawford, M.P. (1966) *The legacy of Nightingale,* p.97. Welsh Regional Hospital Board, Welsh Hospital Staff Committee.

Dan Mason Research Committee (1956) *The work of recently qualified nurses,* (a) p. 34 (b) p.35. London: Dan Mason Research Committee.

Dan Mason Research Committee (1960) *The work, responsibilities and status of the staff nurse,* (a) p.16 (b) p.13 (c) p.69. London: Dan Mason Research Committee.

Garrett, H.E. (1958) *Statistics in psychology and education,* (a) p.278 (b) p.53 (c) p.372 (d) p.142 (e) pp.175-176. New York, London, Toronto: Longman.

Geddes, J.D.C. (1968) Clinical instructors: looking back. *Nursing Times,* **64**, No. 42, 1404-1405.

General Nursing Council for Scotland (1970) *Annual Report, 1970,* p.7. Edinburgh: General Nursing Council for Scotland.

General Nursing Council for Scotland (1970) *Suggested revision of training for the registers,* p.4. (Unpublished).

Hockey, L. (1966) *Feeling the pulse.* London: Queen's Institute of District Nursing.

Home Department (1968) *Report of the Committee on Local Authority and Allied Personal Social Services*, presented to Parliament by the Secretary of State for the Home Department, the Secretary of State for Education and Science, the Minister of Housing and Local Government and the Minister of Health... Cmnd. 3703. London: H.M.S.O.

Lancaster, A. (1971) *The Nurse Teacher: Preparation for a Changing Role?* (a) p.30 (b) p.31. Report submitted to the General Nursing Council for Scotland. (Unpublished). Published (1972) *Nurse Teacher. The Report of an Opinion Survey.* Edinburgh: Churchill Livingstone.

Lancet (1932) *The Lancet Commission on Nursing.* (a) pp.62-63 (b) p.68 London: *Lancet.*

Lancet (1970) Adding drugs to intravenous infusions. (Leading article) ii, 556-557.

Lancet (1970) Doctor and nurse. (Leading article) ii, 971-972.

Lancet (1971) Teaching asepsis to students. (Leading article) i, 639-640.

Lewis, D.G. (1967) *Statistical methods in education*, p.104. University of London Press.

Lord, W.J.H. (1965) The general practitioner, the social worker and the health visitor. *Journal of the College of General Practitioners*, **10**, 247-256.

MacGuire, J. (1969) *Threshold to nursing*, p.84. London: Bell.

Marsh, G.N. (1969) Visiting nurse—analysis to one year's work. *British Medical Journal*, vi, 42-44.

Ministry of Health, Scottish Home and Health Department (1966) *The report of the Committee on Senior Nursing Staff Structure*, p.172. London: H.M.S.O.

Ministry of Health, Department of Health for Scotland, Ministry of Labour and National Service (1947) *Report of the Working Party on the Recruitment and Training of Nurses*, (a) p.43 (b) p.43 (c) p.20 (d) p.60 (e) p.28. London: H.M.S.O.

Nuffield Provincial Hospitals Trust (1953) *The work of nurses in hospital wards*, (a) p.38 (b) p.107 (c) p.145 (d) p.145 (e) p.146 (f) p.138. London: Nuffield Provincial Hospitals Trust.

Oakeshott, M. (1967) Learning and teaching, *in* Peters, R.S. *the Concept of Education,* (a) p.164 (b) p.165 (c) pp. 167-168. London: Routledge and Kegan Paul.

Otis, A.S. (n.d.) *Manual of directions and key for Intermediate and Higher Examinations*, (a) p.1 (b) p.3. London: Harrap.

Oxford Area Nurse Training Committee (1966) *From student to nurse,* (a) p.51 (b) p.42 (c) p.24. Oxford Area Nurse Training Committee.

Pickering, G. (1971) Medicine and society—past, present and future. *British Medical Journal*, i, 191-196.

Royal College of General Practitioners (1968) *The practice nurse*, p.22. London: Royal College of General Practitioners.

Royal College of Nursing (1943) *Nursing Reconstruction Committee report*, Section II Education and Training, Section III Recruitment, (a) p.7 (b) p.12. London: Royal College of Nursing.

Scott, R. (1965) Medicine in society. *Journal of the College of General Practitioners*, **9**, 3-16.

Scott Wright, M. (1961) *A study of the performance of student nurses in relation to a new method of training*, with special reference to the evaluation of an experimental course of basic nursing education being conducted in Scotland, p.269. Ph.D. Thesis, University of Edinburgh.

Scott Wright, M. (1968) *Student nurses in Scotland: characteristics of success and failure,* (a) p.3 (b) p.33 (c) p.35. Scottish Health Service Studies No. 7. Edinburgh: Scottish Home and Health Department.

Secretary of State for Social Security, Secretary of State for Scotland, Secretary of State for Wales (1972) *Report of the Committee on Nursing.* Cmnd. 5115. London: H.M.S.O.

Sexton, K. (1970) Reforming nursing education. (Correspondence) *Nursing Times*, **66**, No. 42, 1318-1319.

Sim, M. (1970) Seebohm sequel. (Correspondence) *British Medical Journal*, iv, 685.

Statutory Instruments (1962) *The Nurses (Scotland) (Amendment) Rules 1962*, Approval Instrument 1962, No. 2195 (S.104). H.M.S.O.

Statutory Instruments (1970) *The Nurses (Scotland) Rules 1970,* No. 1737 (S. 141), p.9. H.M.S.O.

Super, M.A. & Crites, J.O. (1965) *Appraising educational fitness,* (a) p.104 (b) p.104. New York, London: Harper & Row.

Vernon, P.E. (1956) *The measurement of abilities,* 2nd edn., (a) p.222 (b) p.221 footnote.

Watkins, B. (1964) *Bedside teaching,* p.16. London: Nursing Mirror.

Weston Smith, J. & Mottram, E.M. (1967) General practice observed: extended use of nursing services in general practice. *British Medical Journal,* iv, 672-674.

Weston Smith, J. & O'Donovan, J.B. (1970) General practice observed: the practice nurse—a new look. *British Medical Journal,* iv, 673-677.

World Health Organization (1956) *Basic nursing curriculum in Europe,* (a) p.21 (b) p.20. Geneva: World Health Organization.

Wright, M. Scott, *see* Scott Wright, M.

BIBLIOGRAPHY

Albert, A. (1960) *Selective Toxicity*, 2nd edn. London: Methuen.
Anderson, B.E. (1966) *Nursing Education in Junior Colleges*. Philadelphia: Lippincott.
Bell, G.H., Davidson, J.N. & Scarborough, H. (1959) *Textbook of Physiology and Biochemistry*,, 4th edn. Edinburgh: Livingstone.
Bridgman, M. (1955) *Collegiate Education for Nursing*. New York: Russell Sage Foundation.
British Medical Association & Pharmaceutical Society of Great Britain (1959) *British National Formulary 1957 Alternative Edition*. London: British Medical Association.
Brown, E.L. (1948) *Nursing for the Future*. New York: Russell Sage Foundation.
Burling, T., Lentz, E.M. & Wilson, R.N. (1956) *Give and Take in Hospitals*. New York: Putnam's.
Cruickshank, R. ed. (1962) *Mackie and McCartney's Handbook of Bacteriology*, 10th edn. Edinburgh: Livingstone.
Davidson, S. (1962) *Principles and Practice of Medicine*, 6th edn. Edinburgh: Livingstone.
Department of Health and Social Security (1969) *Nursing attachments to General Practice*. London: H.M.S.O.
Ehret, W.F. (1947) *General Chemistry for Colleges*, 6th edn. London: Bell.
Guyton, A.C. (1959) *Functions of the Human Body*. London: Saunders.
Harmer, B. & Henderson, V. (1960) *Textbook of the principles and Practice of Nursing*, 5th edn. New York- Macmillan.
Hector, W. (1962) *Modern Nursing Theory and Practice*, 2nd edn. London: Heinemann.
Hill, A.B. (1961) *Principles of Medical Statistics*, 7th edn. New York: Oxford University Press.
Hill, W.F. (1964) *Learning*. London: Methuen.
Hunter, I.M. (1957), *Memory: Facts and Fallacies*. Harmondsworth: Penguin.
Institute for Social Research (1967 *A Comprehensive Medical School*. London: Institute for Social Research.
Lamberton, E.C. (1958) *Education for Nursing Leadership* Philadelphia: Lippincott.
Micheels, W.J. & Karnes, M.R. (1950) *Measuring Educational Achievement*. London: McGraw-Hill.
Montag, M.L. (1959) *Community College Education for Nursing*. New York: McGraw-Hill.
Moroney, J. (1962) *Surgery for Nurses*, 8th edn. Edinburgh: Livingstone.
Nash, D.F.E. (1961) *The Principles and Practice of Surgical Nursing*, 2nd edn. London: Arnold.
Noakes, G.R. (1957) *New Intermediate Physics*. London: Macmillan.
Richardson, E. (1967) *Group Study for Teachers*. London: Routledge & Kegan Paul.
Ross, J.S. & Wilson, K.J.W. (1957) *Foundations of Nursing*, 2nd ed. Edinburgh: Livingstone.
Royal College of Nursing (1956) *Observations and Objectives* London: Royal College of Nursing.

Royal College of Nursing and National Council of Nurses of the United Kingdom (1964). *A reform of Nursing Education.* London: Royal College of Nursing and National Council of Nurses of the United Kingdom.

Royal Commission on Medical Education (1968) *Report Presented to Parliament...* Cmnd. 3569. London: H.M.S.O.

Skipper, J.K. & Leonard, R.C. (1965), *Social Interaction and Patient Care.* Philadelphia: Lippincott.

Toohey, M. (1962) *Medicine for Nurses,,* 5th edn. Edinburgh: Livingstone.

Vernon, P.E. (1950) *The Structure of Human Abilities.* London: Methuen.

Walton, H.J. (1970) *Professional Education in the University: Medicine—Art or Science.* Seminar on Higher Education in the Seventies, University of Edinburgh. (Unpublished).

Williams, R.E.O., Blowers, R., Garrod, L.P. & Shooter, R.A. (1966) *Hospital Infection,* 2nd edn. London: Lloyd-Luke.

Wilson, A. & Schild, H.O. (1959) *Applied Pharmacology (Clark)* 9th edn. London: Churchill.

World Health Organization (1950) *Expert Committee on Professional and Technical Education of Medical and Auxiliary Personnel.* Technical Report Series No. 22. Geneva: World Health Organization.

World Health Organization (1953) *Working conference on Nursing Education.* Technical Report Series No. 60. Geneva: World Health Organization.